Fast Facts

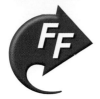

D0232048

Fast Facts:
Colorectal Cancer

Third edition

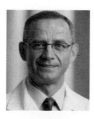

Irving Taylor MD ChM FRCS FMedSci
Professor of Surgery
Director of Medical Studies and Vice Dean
UCL Medical School
University College London
London, UK

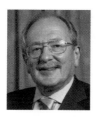

Julio Garcia-Aguilar MD PhD
Professor of Surgery
Chair, Department of Surgery
City of Hope
Duarte, California, USA

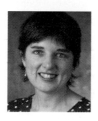

Robyn Ward MBBS PhD FRACP
Director of Area Cancer Services
South East Sydney and Illawarra Area Health Service
Professor of Medicine
POW Clinical School
The University of New South Wales
Sydney, Australia

Declaration of Independence
This book is as balanced and as practical as we can make it.
Ideas for improvement are always welcome: feedback@fastfacts.com

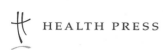

HEALTH PRESS

Fast Facts: Colorectal Cancer
First published 1999; second edition 2002
Third edition February 2010

Text © 2010 Irving Taylor, Julio Garcia-Aguilar, Robyn Ward
© 2010 in this edition Health Press Limited
Health Press Limited, Elizabeth House, Queen Street, Abingdon,
Oxford OX14 3LN, UK
Tel: +44 (0)1235 523233
Fax: +44 (0)1235 523238

Book orders can be placed by telephone or via the website.
For regional distributors or to order via the website, please go to:
www.fastfacts.com
For telephone orders, please call +44 (0)1752 202301 (UK and Europe),
1 800 247 6553 (USA, toll free), +1 419 281 1802 (Americas) or
+61 (0)2 9698 7755 (Asia–Pacific).

Fast Facts is a trademark of Health Press Limited.

A CIP record for this title is available from the British Library.

ISBN 978-1-905832-02-6

Taylor I (Irving)
Fast Facts: Colorectal Cancer/
Irving Taylor, Julio Garcia-Aguilar, Robyn Ward

Medical illustrations by Dee McLean, London, UK.
Typesetting and page layout by Zed, Oxford, UK.
Printed by Latimer Trend & Company Limited, Plymouth, UK.

Text printed on biodegradable and recyclable
paper manufactured using elemental chlorine free (ECF)
wood pulp from well-managed forests.

FSC

Mixed Sources
Product group from well-managed
forests and other controlled sources

Cert no. SGS-COC-005493
www.fsc.org
© 1996 Forest Stewardship Council

Glossary

Adenocarcinoma: a malignant tumor of epithelial origin that is derived from glandular tissue

Adenoma: a benign tumor of epithelial origin that is derived from glandular tissue; an adenoma may undergo malignant change to become an adenocarcinoma

Amsterdam criteria: clinical diagnostic criteria, established to identify families with a highly penetrant dominant form of colorectal cancer (Amsterdam criteria I); the criteria were later modified to include extracolonic tumors (Amsterdam criteria II). These families were previously described as having hereditary non-polyposis colorectal cancer (HNPCC). Nowadays, families who meet Amsterdam criteria are subdivided into those with a germline mutation in the mismatch repair (MMR) genes (Lynch syndrome) or those who do not show abrogation of the MMR pathway (familial colorectal cancer syndrome X)

APC: abbreviation for the *adenomatous polyposis coli* gene, which is responsible for the development of familial adenomatous polyposis (FAP)

Astler–Coller staging system: version of the Dukes classification for colorectal cancer that takes into account spread through the bowel wall and the involvement of proximal and distal lymph nodes

CTC: computed tomography colonography; a method used to visualize the bowel, involving thin-section helical computed tomography of the prepared bowel followed by three-dimensional reconstruction

Differentiation: the degree of similarity of tumor architecture to the structure of the organ from which the tumor arose

Diverticular disease: a condition in which there are diverticula (explained below) in the colon, which give rise to abdominal pain and disturbed bowel habit; the pain is due to muscle spasm, not inflammation

Diverticulitis: inflammation of colonic diverticula, often caused by infection; causes lower abdominal pain with diarrhea or constipation

Diverticulum: a pouch or sac that forms at weak points in the walls of the gastrointestinal tract; may be caused by increased pressure from within, or pulling from outside the tract

Dukes staging: the established system for defining colorectal cancer risk groups; tumors are graded A to C (*see* 'Modified Dukes staging')

Epigenetic changes: heritable (from cell to cell) changes that regulate gene expression but do not affect the DNA sequence. The two main types of epigenetic phenomena are DNA methylation and histone modification, which affect gene transcription and expression by complex and interrelated mechanisms

FAP: familial adenomatous polyposis, an autosomal dominant condition in which thousands of polyps develop in the colon in the teens and early twenties and ultimately lead to malignancy in the fourth or fifth decade

FIT: fecal immunochemical test

FOBT: fecal occult blood test

Hamartoma: an overgrowth of mature tissue, the elements of which are arranged in a disordered fashion and out of proportion compared with the normal tissue; hamartomas are usually benign, but malignancy may occur within the individual tissues

HNPCC: hereditary non-polyposis colorectal cancer, a hereditary syndrome due to a mutation of the mismatch repair (MMR) genes, characterized by the familial clustering of early-onset colorectal cancer and extracolonic cancers; synonymous with Lynch syndrome

Lynch syndrome: an autosomal dominant predisposition to colorectal, endometrial, gastric, ovarian and transitional cell cancers. Lynch syndrome I applies to families with colorectal cancers only; Lynch syndrome II applies to families with colorectal and extracolonic cancers

Malignant ascites: accumulation of fluid in the peritoneal cavity, causing swelling of the abdomen

Mesorectal resection: radical surgical treatment of rectal cancer to avoid the risk of recurrence; the rectum is removed en bloc with the mesorectum

Mesorectum: the mesenteric fat surrounding the rectum that harbors the blood vessels and lymphatics

Metastasis: the distant spread of a malignant tumor from its site of origin; the liver is the most common site of metastatic spread in colorectal cancer

MMR: mismatch repair, a family of genes encoding proteins that repair mismatches that normally occur during DNA replication; includes the *MSH2*, *MLH1*, *MSH6* and *PMS2* genes

Modified Dukes staging: an extension of the traditional Dukes staging (*see* 'Dukes staging') that takes into account spread through the bowel wall and the involvement of proximal and distal lymph nodes; in contrast to the original Dukes staging, tumors can be graded A to D, where D represents metastatic disease

Obstipation: severe or complete constipation

PET/CT: positron emission tomography combined with computed tomography

Pneumatosis coli: the presence of numerous gas-filled cysts in the bowel wall; a rare condition

Pneumaturia: presence in the urine of bubbles of air or another gas; may be the result of a fistula between the urinary tract and bowel, the gas coming from colonic bacteria

Pneumoperitoneum: air or gas in the peritoneal cavity

Polyp: a benign growth protruding from a mucous membrane

Tenesmus: continuous or frequently recurring sensation of the desire to defecate but without the production of significant amounts of feces (blood or mucus may be passed)

TNM: tumor–node–metastases system for the classification of tumors, which gives an indication of the extent of spread. The TNM staging system is sponsored by the International Union Against Cancer (UICC) and the American Joint Committee on Cancer (AJCC) and has become the preferred staging system worldwide

Undifferentiated: cells that have lost normal cell characteristics and differentiation to such an extent that it is impossible to define the origin of the cell; typical of rapidly growing malignant tumors

Volvulus: twisting of part of the gastrointestinal tract, which may lead to partial or complete obstruction

Introduction

Colorectal cancer remains one of the most common malignancies affecting Western populations. Many of the genetic and environmental factors that contribute to the development of this disease are now well recognized. Eventually this information will be used to better target prevention and treatment strategies. In the meantime, awareness and prompt investigation of the symptoms associated with colorectal cancer remain a high priority.

Early diagnosis and appropriate surgical therapy are essential to achieve the best chance of cure. Unfortunately, diagnosis is often delayed because of the vagueness of symptoms and patients' reticence to talk about their bowel habits. In addition, health professionals often fail to realize the significance of the patient's symptoms.

Patients should be referred for investigation and treatment at the earliest opportunity. Surgical treatment is often curative when carried out for localized disease. Once metastases have occurred, however, the prognosis is poor and palliation may be the only option. Recent therapeutic developments have changed the way colorectal cancer is treated in both the adjuvant and metastatic setting. In addition to more effective chemotherapeutic agents, new biologic therapies such as the monoclonal antibodies bevacizumab and cetuximab have been introduced into the treatment paradigm.

Despite the impact of new drug therapies, the best opportunities for improving survival from this disease lie in early detection. Improved methodologies for screening asymptomatic populations and also high-risk patient groups are therefore extremely important.

The primary care provider is key in the diagnosis and overall management of patients with colorectal cancer. This new edition of *Fast Facts: Colorectal Cancer* delivers, concisely, the important information required to give an optimal service to patients with this common disease.

Carcinoma of the large bowel – colorectal cancer – is one of the major malignancies in the western world. In the UK, there are more than 36 000 cases each year, with a predominance of men over women, and the disease accounts for some 18 000 deaths. The incidence in the UK has changed little over the last 10 years. Within the UK, the rate of colon cancer is higher in Scotland than in either England or Wales.

In the USA, colorectal cancer is the third most common cancer in both men and women. Incidence in both black and white US men and women gradually increased through most of the 1970s and 1980s. In recent years, incidence in black people has overtaken that in white people. Between 1985 and 2005, there were declines in incidence in all US ethnic populations (Figure 1.1). As of 2004, the latest year for which updated statistics are available, approximately 48 cases of colorectal cancer were diagnosed per 100 000 people. The incidence

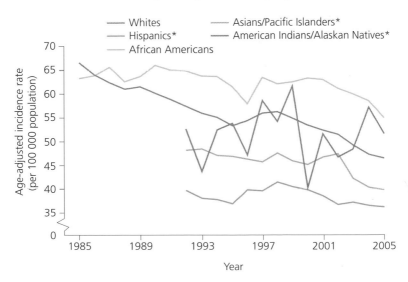

Figure 1.1 Incidence of colorectal cancer in different ethnic populations in the USA. *Data not available before 1992. Adapted from US National Cancer Institute statistics, updated 2008.

of colorectal cancer decreased by almost 26% between 1984 and 2004.

Worldwide, the incidence of colorectal cancer varies widely, with a 20-fold variation between different countries for colon cancer and a 10-fold variation for rectal cancer (Figure 1.2). Incidence of colorectal cancer is apparently lowest in African and Asian countries. The tendency for migrational convergence to occur is now widely recognized, indicating the importance of recent environmental change.

The incidence of colorectal cancer increases with age (Figure 1.3). In the UK, the lifetime risk of being diagnosed with colorectal cancer is 1 in 16 for men and 1 in 20 for women.

The distribution of cancers through the colon also varies. Tumors on the left side of the colon are common, with tumors of the sigmoid colon,

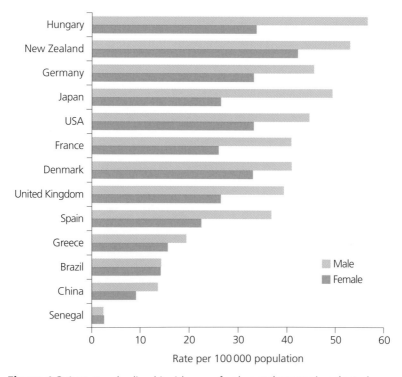

Figure 1.2 Age-standardized incidence of colorectal cancer in selected countries (2002 estimates). Reproduced with permission of Cancer Research UK.

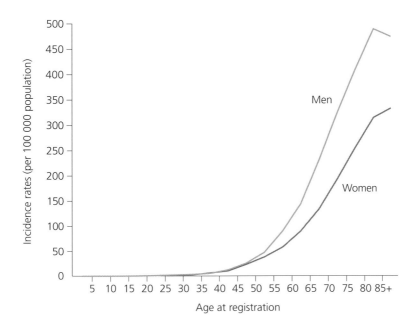

Figure 1.3 Incidence of colorectal cancer by age in men and women in the UK, 2006. Reproduced with permission of Cancer Research UK.

rectosigmoid junction and rectum accounting for nearly 70% of cases worldwide (Figure 1.4). The proportion of right-sided colorectal cancers increases with age. Interestingly, many studies have now reported an increasing incidence of right-sided colon cancer in both sexes in Western countries.

Risk factors

The development of colorectal cancer is thought to be a multifactorial process, involving genetic and environmental factors.

Genetic factors. Colorectal cancer arises from multi-step genetic and epigenetic alterations in oncogenes and tumor suppressor genes. Broadly speaking there are two distinct pathways through which colorectal cancer develops: 85% of cancers develop through the chromosomal instability pathway, characterized by chromosomal losses and gains, while the remaining 15% follow the microsatellite

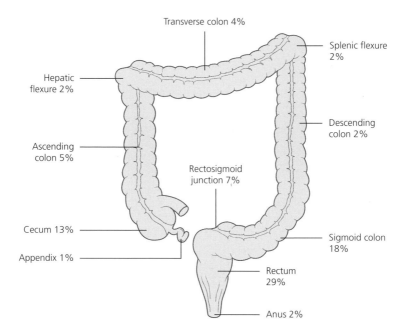

Figure 1.4 Distribution of cases of colorectal cancer within the large bowel and rectum (a further 15% of cases are unspecified). Note the higher incidence on the left side. (Based on data from England, 1997–2000.) Reproduced with permission of Cancer Research UK.

instability pathway, which is caused by a failure of mismatch repair, usually because the *MLH1* gene is inactivated (Figure 1.5).

Rarely, some individuals are born with an inherited predisposition to develop colorectal cancer. The three well-known inherited conditions are:

- familial adenomatous polyposis (FAP), caused by a germline mutation in the *adenomatous polyposis coli* (*APC*) gene
- Lynch syndrome, caused by a germline mutation in one of the mismatch repair (MMR) genes
- MYH-associated polyposis, an autosomal recessive condition caused by germline mutations in the *MYH* gene.

In FAP, thousands of polyps occur throughout the colon, and malignancy will develop inevitably unless the colon is removed. Lynch syndrome is characterized by early-onset colorectal cancer as well as

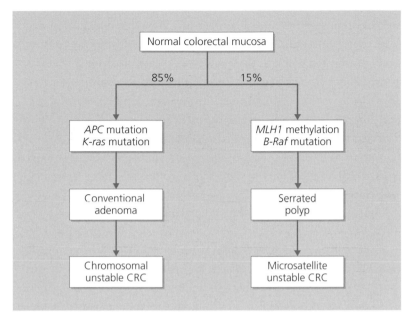

Figure 1.5 A model for the development of colorectal cancer (CRC) showing the chromosomal instability and microsatellite instability pathways. The common morphologic, genetic and epigenetic changes are also shown. Serrated polyp refers to a hyperplastic polyp or serrated adenoma. Gene mutations responsible for the development of colorectal cancer include *APC*, *B-Raf*, *K-ras* and *MLH1*.

extracolonic cancers (see pages 40–1), including cancers of the upper gastrointestinal tract, urinary tract and female genital tract. Lynch syndrome accounts for 2–5% of all colorectal cancers.

In addition, 25% of patients with colorectal cancer have a family history of the disease or polyps, suggesting a hereditary predisposition. The genetics of these families are being investigated.

Environmental factors. There is much evidence linking the 'Western' diet (high fat and low fiber content) to the development of colorectal cancer. Other environmental factors that may be involved include a high alcohol intake (particularly beer) and obesity. Any linkage with fat intake is still unclear and is probably related to meat intake. Although it is difficult to interpret dietary studies, there is evidence that a healthy well-balanced diet that is high in fiber and low in fat and alcohol may offer some protection. A number of possible dietary influences have been investigated (Table 1.1). An extensive study involving 149 000 participants has suggested an increased incidence of colon cancer (30–40% more likely) in patients who consume large amounts of red and processed meats over a long period of time.

Interestingly, migrant studies have demonstrated that people who move from low- to high-incidence areas (e.g. Japanese who have moved to the USA) also develop the high rates of colorectal cancer associated with their host country.

There is some suggestion that a high calcium intake reduces epithelial proliferation in the gastrointestinal tract, though there is little evidence that calcium in high doses is protective. The Women's Health Initiative trial reported that calcium and vitamin D did not have any protective effect. Other vitamins are thought to have a role in inhibiting malignant transformation by affecting the antioxidants present within the colon.

Case–control studies have consistently shown a protective effect of aspirin (even at low doses taken for cardiovascular benefit) and other non-steroidal anti-inflammatory drugs on colorectal cancer. However, in view of the known side effects of these drugs, it is premature to recommend their widespread use as chemoprotective agents.

The relationship between colorectal cancer and inflammatory bowel disease is discussed in detail in Chapter 4.

TABLE 1.1

Possible dietary factors in colorectal cancer risk

Factor	Examples	Effect
Antioxidants	Vitamins E and C	Protective
Micronutrients	Calcium, folic acid	Protective
Macronutrients	Fat	Promoter
	Fiber	Protective
Food mutagens	Heterocyclic amines	Promoter

Histological features

Colorectal cancer is an adenocarcinoma arising from the epithelial lining of the bowel. Some colorectal cancers may develop de novo, but most result from malignant transformation of adenomatous polyps. There are four types of polyp that are thought to give rise to cancer:

- tubular adenomas
- villous adenomas
- tubulovillous adenomas
- serrated polyps (includes serrated and sessile serrated adenomas).

Polyps arise from the mucosa and gradually increase in size. Some polyp characteristics – size larger than 1 cm, tubulovillous or villous histology, multiple occurrences – are associated with a high risk of malignant transformation. Most screening programs are designed to recognize the presence of polyps, or early malignant change in polyps or surrounding mucosa (Figure 1.6).

Staging classifications

Dukes staging from 1932 was the first system used to describe colorectal cancer risk groups:

- Dukes A – confined to the bowel wall
- Dukes B – involving the full thickness of the bowel wall to the serosa
- Dukes C – involvement of mesenteric lymph nodes.

The modified Dukes staging and Astler–Coller staging systems are versions of the Dukes classification that take into account spread

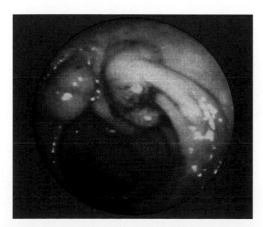

Figure 1.6 Colonoscopic appearance of polyps within the colon showing one polyp on a stalk (pedunculated).

through the bowel wall, the involvement of proximal and distal lymph nodes and the presence of distant metastases (Dukes D).

More recently, the tumor–nodes–metastases (TNM) classification of colorectal cancer, which gives an indication of the extent of spread, has become established as the preferred staging system (Table 1.2). This

---

TABLE 1.2

Tumor–Nodes–Metastases (TNM) classification of colorectal cancer

Primary tumor (T)
Pathological staging

TX   Primary tumor cannot be assessed

T0   No evidence of primary tumor

Tis   Carcinoma in situ: intraepithelial or invasion of lamina propria*

T1   Tumor invades submucosa

T2   Tumor invades muscularis propria

T3   Tumor invades through the muscularis propria into the subserosa, or into non-peritonealized pericolic or perirectal tissues

T4   Tumor directly invades other organs or structures, and/or perforates visceral peritoneum†

Ultrasound staging

uT0 Benign tumor

uT1 Invasion into but not through the submucosa

uT2 Invasion into but not through the muscularis propria

uT3 Invasion into perirectal fat

uT4 Invasion into adjacent organs

*Tis includes cancer cells confined within the glandular basement membrane (intraepithelial) or lamina propria (intramucosal) with no extension through the muscularis mucosa into the submucosa.
†Direct invasion in T4 includes invasion of other segments of the colorectum by way of the serosa (e.g. invasion of the sigmoid colon by a carcinoma of the cecum).

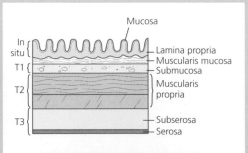

A cross-section through the bowel wall illustrating the primary tumor (T) section of the TNM classification.

classification is important for colon and rectal cancers of all stages, but becomes particularly important in rectal cancer when local therapies, rather than major ablative surgery, are being considered (e.g. for a T1 or T2 tumor).

Regional lymph nodes (N)

NX   Regional lymph nodes cannot be assessed

N0   No regional lymph node metastasis

N1   Metastases in 1–3 regional lymph nodes

N2   Metastases in 4 or more regional lymph nodes

uN0 No metastatic perirectal node

uN1 Metastatic perirectal nodes

Distant metastases (M)

MX   Distant metastases cannot be assessed

M0   No distant metastases

M1   Distant metastases

Stage grouping

AJCC/UICC[‡]				Dukes[§]
Stage 0	Tis	N0	M0	–
Stage I	T1	N0	M0	A
	T2	N0	M0	–
Stage II	T3	N0	M0	B
	T4	N0	M0	–
Stage III	Any T	N1	M0	C
	Any T	N2	M0	–
Stage IV	Any T	Any N	M1	D

[‡]American Joint Committee on Cancer/International Union Against Cancer.
[§]Dukes B is a composite of better (T3/N0/M0) and worse (T4/N0/M0) prognostic groups, as is Dukes C (any T/N1/M0 and any T/N2/M0).

Prognosis. Dukes and TNM staging are also important for determining prognosis. Patients with stage I colorectal cancer have an excellent prognosis, whereas those with stage III have a much worse prognosis (Figure 1.7). Unfortunately, the incidence of stage I colorectal cancer is less than 10%, compared with 45% for stage III disease. Approximately 20% of patients present with stage IV colorectal cancer, few of whom survive for 5 years. In addition to tumor stage, prognosis is estimated by examining the following characteristics:

- the presence of tumor in lymphovascular vessels
- the number of lymph nodes retrieved at resection (12 or more is optimal)
- whether the margins of the resection specimen are clear of tumor.

The degree of differentiation of colorectal cancer may also be important in determining prognosis. Unfortunately, however, this parameter is often inconsistently reported in pathology reports and it may not be reliable.

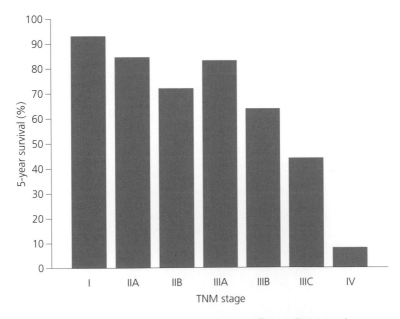

Figure 1.7 Prognosis for colorectal cancer according to TNM staging. TNM, tumor–nodes–metastases (see Table 1.2). Data from the US National Cancer Institute Surveillance and End Results (SEER) database.

Tumors are divided into: well differentiated, moderately differentiated, poorly differentiated and undifferentiated. A well-differentiated tumor will have a relatively good prognosis whereas the undifferentiated state is typical of a rapidly growing, malignant tumor.

Pattern of spread

Large bowel cancer is locally invasive, spreading through the full thickness of the bowel wall into adjacent tissues. Symptoms of obstruction occur as the lumen of the bowel is occluded (Chapter 6). Unfortunately, however, metastatic spread may be evident before local growth produces symptoms.

The most common site of metastases is the liver. Approximately 20% of patients have liver metastases at the time of colorectal resection, and approximately 30% of all other patients will subsequently develop liver metastases (Chapter 7). Other sites of metastatic spread are the lungs, brain and bones, but these are unusual in the absence of liver metastases. Patients may also develop peritoneal spread with the formation of malignant ascites.

Prognosis is significantly better when colorectal cancer is diagnosed and treated at an early stage. The disease tends to progress in a predictable manner from benign to malignant lesions, and then to metastatic spread. Clearly, it is far better to treat a patient early, with the expectation of cure, than to manage the serious effects of metastatic involvement.

Key points – epidemiology and pathophysiology

- Colorectal cancer is one of the major malignancies in the Western world.
- The lifetime incidence in the UK is 1 in 16 for men and 1 in 20 for women.
- Both environmental and genetic factors are responsible.
- Prognosis depends on the extent of spread at diagnosis.
- Polyps are frequently pre-malignant.

Key references

Boyle P, Leon ME. Epidemiology of colorectal cancer. *Br Med Bull* 2002;64:1–25.

Dunlop MG, Farrington SM, Carothers AD et al. Cancer risk associated with germline DNA mismatch repair gene mutations. *Hum Mol Genet* 1997;6:105–10.

EUCAN (European Network of Cancer Registries). Cancer incidence, mortality and prevalence in the European Union. 2001.

Jackson-Thompson J, Ahmed F, German RR et al. Descriptive epidemiology of colorectal cancer in the United States, 1998–2001. *Cancer* 2006;107(5 Suppl):1103–11.

Keating J, Pater P, Lolohea S, Wickremesekera K. The epidemiology of colorectal cancer: what can we learn from the New Zealand Cancer registry? *N Z Med J* 2003;116:U437.

Terry P, Giovannucci E, Michels KB et al. Fruit, vegetables, dietary fiber, and risk of colorectal cancer. *J Natl Cancer Inst* 2001;93:525–33.

Wei EK, Giovannucci E, Wu K et al. Comparison of risk factors for colon and rectal cancer. *Int J Cancer* 2004; 108:433–42.

A detailed history and examination will often reveal the site of malignancy within the large bowel or rectum. Patients with colorectal cancer can develop a myriad of symptoms, as highlighted below.

Abdominal pain

Frequently, abdominal pain is non-specific and may be localized to any quadrant of the abdomen or may be diffuse. When the pain is persistent and colicky, it is more likely to represent obstructive symptoms resulting from a lesion in the descending colon. More localized tenderness with signs of localized peritonitis indicates local invasion of the adjacent peritoneum. It is uncommon for colorectal cancer to perforate the bowel, but when it does the prognosis is significantly worse. Patients with persistent perineal pain associated with tenesmus are more likely to have a large rectal cancer. It can be difficult to distinguish the pain associated with diverticular disease from that due to a carcinoma in the sigmoid or descending colon. Patients with diverticular disease can also have an underlying carcinoma; investigation of this patient group is therefore important.

It should be remembered that the presence of colon cancer can be brought to light as a result of investigations for other suspected pathology. For example, biliary colic due to gallstones may be demonstrated on ultrasound scan but the possibility of the symptoms being due to another pathology such as colon cancer should also be considered.

Change in bowel habit

Any patient over 45 years of age who presents with an alteration in bowel habit that lasts for more than 2 weeks should probably be investigated. The change in bowel habit might be diarrhea, which may be bloody, possibly associated with a sense of incomplete defecation. Patients frequently complain of diarrhea when they are actually suffering from incomplete defecation, a symptom often associated with tenesmus. These latter symptoms indicate a rectal tumor. Patients with constipation and associated colicky abdominal pain may have an underlying obstructive lesion and should be investigated.

Alternating diarrhea and constipation associated with colicky abdominal pain is uncommon; this indicates a subacute obstruction of the large bowel.

Rectal bleeding

Rectal bleeding is common and is often associated with hemorrhoids. Blood from hemorrhoids is usually bright red and is accompanied by anal discomfort. The bleeding is intermittent and splashes the toilet pan.

Rectal blood that is darker in color and mixed in with stool is more likely to be secondary to an underlying carcinoma. Rectal bleeding associated with tenesmus should be investigated urgently. Patients who have recently developed rectal bleeding should be examined carefully, particularly if over 45 years of age, to exclude the presence of an underlying rectal tumor. Rectal bleeding always demands diagnostic investigation.

Anemia

The development of non-specific anemia of 'unknown origin' is not uncommon in patients with a carcinoma in the ascending colon. As these patients rarely have abdominal pain, they generally present with advanced disease. Bleeding is occult and may be recognized on a fecal occult blood test (see pages 34–6). The anemia is iron deficient and microcytic. In the UK, the initial investigation of such patients is often by gastroscopy, as an upper gastrointestinal disorder is suspected. If this proves normal, the next most logical investigation is colonoscopy. In the USA, by contrast, patients with non-specific anemia tend to be examined initially with colonoscopy, as carcinoma of the right colon is believed to be 'silent'.

New symptoms

Anorexia and weight loss frequently accompany colorectal cancer and are often associated with advanced disease. The differential diagnosis in these patients is a gastric carcinoma, but when investigations are negative it is important to exclude a large bowel malignancy.

Early diagnosis

The earlier diagnosis is made and treatment initiated, the better the prognosis. In the UK, guidelines have been introduced to highlight specific symptoms that indicate more rapid referral to a specialist team:

- rectal bleeding with a change in bowel habit
- rectal bleeding without anal symptoms
- change in bowel habit, including increased frequency and loose stools for several weeks
- any indication of intestinal obstruction (colicky abdominal pain, distension, constipation).

Examination

Features on clinical examination that should arouse suspicion of malignancy include:

- anemia (hemoglobin < 10 g/dL)
- abdominal mass(es).

A mass in the right iliac fossa indicates extensive cecal or ascending colon carcinoma, whereas a mass in the left iliac fossa indicates sigmoid carcinoma. Rectal examination can reveal a carcinoma of the rectum, and masses may be palpated in the Pouch of Douglas or anteriorly in men. This indicates either a carcinoma within the sigmoid colon or peritoneal metastases within the pelvis.

The degree of fixity of a tumor on rectal examination is important and may have a bearing on subsequent treatment. It is occasionally difficult to distinguish a rectal cancer from a prostate or fixed cervical malignancy, but biopsy should assist in this regard.

It is often possible to distinguish cancers on the right side of the colon from cancers on the left side by means of symptomatology and clinical examination (Table 2.1).

Hepatomegaly indicates advanced disease with extensive liver metastases, and is a harbinger of a very poor prognosis. The usual symptoms of advanced malignancy are anorexia, weight loss, lethargy, and possibly right upper quadrant pain from hepatomegaly. Jaundice is rare, however.

TABLE 2.1

Symptoms of colorectal cancer

Right colon	Left colon
• Little pain	• Often colicky pain
• Weight loss	• Weight loss less common
• Occult bleeding	• Rectal bleeding
• Obstructive symptoms uncommon	• Obstructive symptoms and signs
• Mass in right iliac fossa	• Mass in left iliac fossa
• Change in bowel habit uncommon	• Change in bowel habit is an early symptom
• Higher proportion of Dukes C	• Less advanced disease on presentation

Rarer clinical signs of an underlying colorectal cancer include:

- pneumaturia
- gastrocolic fistula
- ischiorectal or perineal abscesses, which indicate underlying rectal cancer
- deep venous thrombosis.

Differential diagnosis. Careful history and examination can exclude:

- diverticular disease
- irritable bowel syndrome
- inflammatory bowel disease
- local rectal pathology (e.g. hemorrhoids)
- ischemic colitis
- pneumatosis coli.

Nevertheless, further investigation is frequently necessary to provide definitive evidence of an underlying carcinoma.

'Alarm features'. Colorectal cancer can cause a myriad of symptoms and signs, many of which are non-specific and highly prevalent among healthy individuals. To help general practitioners to identify patients with a high probability of colorectal cancer, health organizations have developed guidelines that include a list of 'alarm features' such as rectal bleeding, change in bowel habits or unexplained anemia, which should trigger a referral to a specialist for further investigations. However, it is important to remember that many of the alarm features have a poor sensitivity and specificity for the diagnosis of colorectal carcinoma, and the diagnosis requires a high index of suspicion.

Key points – clinical presentation

- Early diagnosis is important, and referral for persistent symptoms is essential.
- Abdominal pain is often non-specific.
- A change in bowel habit that lasts for more than 2 weeks in a patient over 45 years of age requires investigation.
- Rectal bleeding with a change in bowel habit in patients over 45 years of age requires investigation.
- Anorexia and weight loss can indicate advanced colorectal cancer.

Key references

Armitage N. Colorectal cancer: clinical features and investigations. *Medicine* 2003;31:65–6.

Cleary J, Peters TJ, Sharp D, Hamilton W. Clinical features of colorectal cancer before emergency presentation: a population-based case-control study. *Fam Pract* 2007;24:3–6.

Ford AC, Veldhuyzen van Zanten SJ, Rodgers CC et al. Diagnostic utility of alarm features for colorectal cancer: systematic review and meta-analysis. *Gut* 2008;57:1545–53.

Hamilton W, Round A, Sharp D, Peters TJ. Clinical features of colorectal cancer before diagnosis: a population-based case-control study. *Br J Cancer* 2005;93:399–405.

Majumdar SR, Fletcher RH, Evans AT. How does colorectal cancer present? Symptoms, duration, and clues to location. *Am J Gastroenterol* 1999;94:3039–45.

Panzuto F, Chiriatti A, Bevilacqua S et al. Digestive and Liver Disease and Primary Care Medicine Lazio Group. Symptom-based approach to colorectal cancer: survey of primary care physicians in Italy. *Dig Liver Dis* 2003;35:869–75.

Diagnosis and staging

Confirmation of the diagnosis requires examination of the entire colon. Staging of colorectal cancer requires imaging studies and pathological examination of the resected specimen. Accurate staging is essential to identify patients who may benefit from adjuvant therapy, and for determining prognosis.

Diagnosis of the primary tumor

Any patient with a clinical history suggesting colorectal cancer should undergo examination of the entire colon. The goal is to diagnose the primary lesion and to exclude any synchronous polyps or cancers. Traditionally, this has been accomplished by colonoscopy or barium enema.

Colonoscopy provides high-resolution images of the lesion (Figure 3.1) and allows diagnostic (biopsy) or therapeutic (polypectomy) interventions. However, colonoscopy is uncomfortable for the patient and requires conscious sedation. It is technically demanding and cannot be completed to the cecum in 10% of patients. Respiratory depression is not uncommon, and colonic perforation occurs in 0.17% of patients.

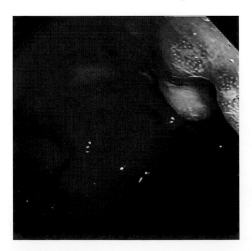

Figure 3.1 Colonoscopy showing carcinoma in the rectum.

Rigid sigmoidoscopy can be used to visualize the rectum and rectosigmoid region, but not the more proximal colon.

In general, colonoscopy is the diagnostic test of choice in most patients suspected of having colorectal cancer.

Double-contrast barium enema is cheaper and safer than colonoscopy, and can image the entire colon in almost 100% of cases. Barium enema is less sensitive than colonoscopy for detecting polyps smaller than 5 mm diameter, but the sensitivity of both techniques is similar for lesions greater than 1 cm diameter (95%). With barium enema, it is not possible to take a biopsy of the tumor or to snare polyps (Figure 3.2).

Double-contrast barium enema should be performed when colonoscopy is not successful in reaching the cecum or in very elderly patients unable to tolerate colonoscopy. This can often be done on the same day, to spare the patient a second bowel preparation.

Enhanced-resolution spiral computed tomography (CT) has enabled CT colonography (CT pneumocolon) to be performed with a high degree of sensitivity and specificity (Figure 3.3). CT pneumocolon can be performed if colonoscopy is not successful for the reasons stated above. Again, it can be undertaken on the same day, to spare the patient a second bowel preparation.

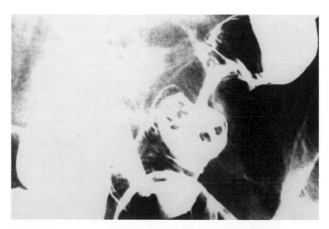

Figure 3.2 Barium enema showing typical carcinoma ('apple-core' stricture, arrowed) in descending colon.

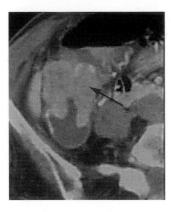

Figure 3.3 Computed tomography pneumocolon demonstrating obstructing carcinoma of the ascending colon.

Diagnosis of metastatic disease

The optimal surgical treatment of colon cancer demands resection of the segment of colon that contains tumor, together with the lymph nodes draining that segment of the bowel. In general, the extent of resection is independent of the stage of the tumor. In order to avoid devastating complications such as large bowel obstruction, hemorrhage or tumor perforation, the primary tumor is sometimes resected, especially left-sided cancers, even if distant metastases are present. However, in patients who have a short life expectancy because of poor general condition or extensive metastatic disease, a non-surgical approach or a less radical resection may be indicated. Non-surgical approaches include the use of colonic stents, which relieve the bowel obstruction without the need for surgery. This strategy is particularly valuable in patients with widespread metastatic disease.

A standard preoperative chest radiograph is useful for the detection of pulmonary metastases. Abdominal CT with contrast should be performed to assess the presence of tumor involvement of adjacent organs, suggesting the need for a more radical resection, or metastatic involvement of the liver (Figure 3.4). The identification of widespread liver or lung metastases in some cases makes resection of the primary tumor an inappropriate treatment choice. Recently, positron emission tomography combined with CT scanning (PET/CT) has been shown to be effective in the recognition of small metastatic deposits, particularly in the liver (Figure 3.5). PET/CT is more sensitive than CT alone for the detection of distant metastases from colorectal cancer.

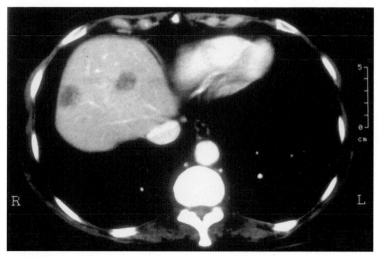

Figure 3.4 CT scan of a primary tumor showing two liver metastases.

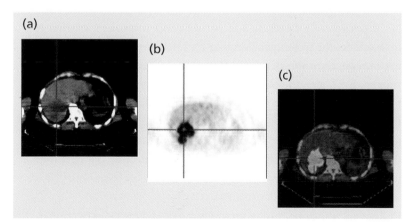

Figure 3.5 (a) Coronal CT scan, (b) PET scan and (c) fused PET/CT image of the liver showing a solitary 'hot spot' representing liver metastasis from a colorectal primary tumor.

Preoperative staging of rectal cancer

In properly selected patients, transanal excision of early rectal cancer results in tumor control equivalent to that obtained with radical surgery, but without the need for major abdominal surgery or a permanent colostomy. However, local excision with curative intent is only appropriate for anatomically accessible tumors that are localized to the bowel wall. A tumor that has spread into the perirectal fat or the regional lymph nodes cannot be cured by local excision alone. Preoperative determination of the depth of mural invasion and the nodal status is therefore critical in selecting patients for local excision. The depth of mural invasion is particularly important because it is directly related to the incidence of lymph node involvement, local recurrence and 5-year survival.

Local and regional staging of rectal cancer relies primarily on four techniques:
- digital rectal examination (DRE)
- endorectal ultrasonography
- magnetic resonance imaging (MRI)
- CT and sometimes PET/CT scan.

Digital rectal examination is only useful for tumors located in the distal portion of the rectum and permits only a gross estimation of invasion depth; accuracy of staging by DRE varies significantly with the experience of the examiner. When correlated with pathological staging, DRE identifies extrarectal invasion with reasonable accuracy but cannot discriminate the degree of intramural invasion. DRE also fails to identify more than 50% of the pathologically proven involved nodes. Thus, DRE is more accurate in staging locally advanced rather than early tumors, and is of limited value in selecting patients for local therapy.

Endorectal ultrasonography provides a 360-degree cross-sectional image of the rectum and perirectal tissue, and can discriminate the different layers of the rectal wall (Figure 3.6). A modification of the tumor–nodes–metastases (TNM) staging system, with degrees of invasion that correspond very closely to the pathological stages, is currently used for preoperative ultrasonographic staging of rectal tumors (see Table 1.2, pages 16–17). Ultrasonographic classification (uT0–uT4) is used in decision making. The accuracy of endorectal ultrasonography is 81–94% for determining the depth of rectal wall invasion, and 58–86% for detecting lymph node metastases.

(a)

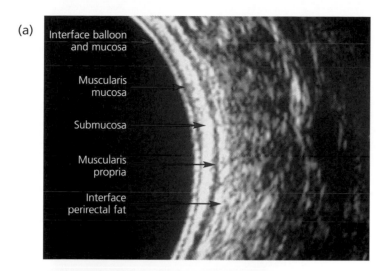

Interface balloon and mucosa

Muscularis mucosa

Submucosa

Muscularis propria

Interface perirectal fat

(b)

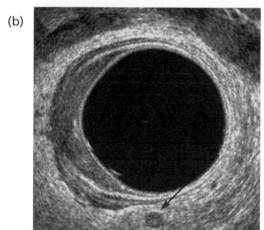

Figure 3.6 Endorectal ultrasound scans: (a) detail of the different layers of the rectal wall; (b) tumor penetrating into the perirectal fat with a metastatic perirectal lymph node (arrowed).

MRI provides excellent cross-sectional images of the rectum, mesorectum and other pelvic structures (Figure 3.7). It is the most accurate imaging modality for assessing the relationship of tumors to the fascia propria of the rectum, which corresponds to the resection margin during standard surgery for rectal cancer. MRI is as accurate as endorectal ultrasonography for detecting nodal metastatic lymph nodes in the mesorectum. MRI is best for selecting patients with advanced tumors who are likely to benefit from adjuvant preoperative treatment. In contrast with endorectal ultrasonography, phased-array MRI does

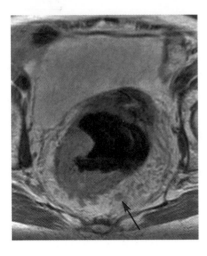

Figure 3.7 MRI scan of the pelvis of a patient with rectal cancer, showing a small perirectal lymph node (arrowed).

not depict the layers of the rectal wall and therefore is not very useful in identifying early rectal cancer that can be treated with local therapy.

CT provides cross-sectional images of the entire abdomen and pelvis and is used routinely in the preoperative evaluation of colon and rectal cancer to assess tumor extension to adjacent organs and to exclude abdominal metastasis. However, its role in the local staging of rectal cancer is limited. As with MRI, CT does not show the layers of the rectal wall and thus is not very useful for staging early rectal cancer. Even the multi-detector row spiral CT scanners are less accurate than phased-array MRI in assessing tumor infiltration of the mesorectal fascia.

Key points – diagnosis and staging

- Early diagnosis is critical.
- Colonoscopy provides visualization and allows biopsy and possibly treatment (polypectomy).
- Patients should have a preoperative CT scan to assess tumor spread.
- MRI is reliable for assessing local invasion of rectal cancer.

PET/CT is used primarily to detect recurrent disease, and is not routinely used for the preoperative staging of rectal cancer. However, there are data suggesting that it may change the preoperative management in 17% of patients.

Key references

Garcia-Aguilar J, Pollack J, Lee SH et al. Accuracy of endorectal ultrasonography in preoperative staging of rectal tumors. *Dis Colon Rectum* 2002;45:10–15.

Gearhart SL, Frassica D, Rosen R et al. Improved staging with pretreatment positron emission tomography/computed tomography in low rectal cancer. *Ann Surg Oncol* 2006;13:397–404.

Hamilton W, Sharp D. Diagnosis of colorectal cancer in primary care: the evidence base for guidelines. *Fam Pract* 2004;21:99–106.

Johnson CD, Chen MH, Toledano AY et al. Accuracy of CT colonography for detection of large adenomas and cancers. *N Engl J Med* 2008;359:1207–17.

Klessen C, Rogalla P, Taupitz M. Local staging of rectal cancer: the current role of MRI. *Eur Radiol* 2007;17:379–89.

MERCURY Study Group. Diagnostic accuracy of preoperative magnetic resonance imaging in predicting curative resection of rectal cancer: prospective observational study. *BMJ* 2006;333:779.

Rex DK, Rahmani EY, Haseman JH et al. Relative sensitivity of colonoscopy and barium enema for detection of colorectal cancer in clinical practice. *Gastroenterology* 1997;112:17–23.

Schaffzin DM, Wong WD. Endorectal ultrasound in the preoperative evaluation of rectal cancer. *Clin Colorectal Cancer* 2004;4:124–32.

Vliegen R, Dresen R, Beets G et al. The accuracy of Multi-detector row CT for the assessment of tumor invasion of the mesorectal fascia in primary rectal cancer. *Abdom Imaging* 2008;33:604–10.

Wolberink SV, Beets-Tan RG, de Haas-Kock DF et al. Conventional CT for the prediction of an involved circumferential resection margin in primary rectal cancer. *Dig Dis* 2007;25:80–5.

Most colorectal cancers develop from benign adenomatous polyps. The accumulation of mutations in oncogenes and tumor suppressor genes over several years (see Chapter 1) can result in the transformation of normal colonic mucosa into an invasive carcinoma. The slow development of colorectal cancer provides a window of opportunity for the detection and removal of premalignant adenomatous polyps and early-stage cancers. Removal of adenomatous polyps reduces the incidence of cancer, and the diagnosis of colorectal cancers at earlier stages reduces mortality.

Screening methods

Fecal tests primarily detect cancer. The tests used are:
- fecal occult blood test (FOBT)
- fecal immunochemical test (FIT)
- stool DNA test.
  Structural examinations detect polyps and cancers. These include:
- sigmoidoscopy
- colonoscopy
- double-contrast barium enema
- computed tomography colonography (CTC).

Fecal occult blood test. Colorectal cancers and polyps bleed more than the normal mucosa. Bleeding is usually intermittent, but the chance of bleeding is proportional to the size of the tumor. Detection of tumor bleeding is the basis of the most widely used screening test: the guaiac-based detection of the pseudoperoxidase activity of hemoglobin in the stool (Figure 4.1). For the FOBT, two samples from three consecutive stools are smeared onto the window of a card that contains the guaiac reagent; a change in color of the reagent indicates the presence of blood (Figure 4.2). Some foods such as red meat, and medications such as acetylsalicylic acid (ASA; aspirin) and non-steroidal anti-inflammatory drugs can cause a false-positive reaction, so a special diet must be

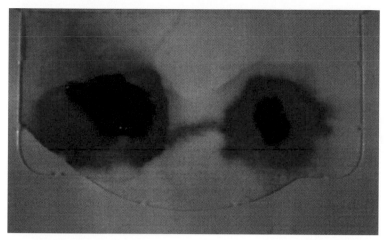

Figure 4.1 Guaiac-based test showing positive result for fecal occult blood.

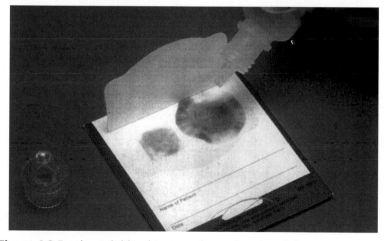

Figure 4.2 Fecal occult blood test – a change in color of the reagent indicates the presence of blood.

followed for 2 or 3 days before the test. Other foods and drugs, in particular vitamin C, can result in false-negative results and should also be avoided for several days before a test.

The FOBT is not specific for cancer; bleeding from any other source in the gastrointestinal tract will give a positive result. As most tumors bleed slowly and intermittently, the sensitivity of the test is low. Methods aimed at increasing the sensitivity, such as rehydrating the cards, reduce the specificity of the test. The sensitivity of the test increases with the number of samples tested; testing of stool samples from several consecutive days is therefore recommended.

Several prospective randomized trials have demonstrated that screening by FOBT followed by total colonic evaluation with colonoscopy in individuals with a positive test reduces the mortality from colorectal cancer.

In England, a national screening program based on FOB testing is offered every 2 years to all men and women aged 60–69 years. Screening centers across the country provide specialist nurse-run clinics for people who receive an abnormal test result, as well as endoscopy facilities. The centers are also responsible for referring those requiring treatment to their local hospital multidisciplinary team. It is anticipated that around 2% of those tested in the UK will have an abnormal result and will need to be referred for further investigation and offered a colonoscopy.

Fecal immunochemical test. The FIT detects human globin in the stool using immunochemical methods. It is as sensitive as the FOBT but is more specific for human blood. It also avoids false-negative results in the presence of vitamin C, and is more specific for lower gastrointestinal bleeding because the globin is degraded by digestive enzymes. It does not require dietary modification before the test, and the handling of the specimens is less demanding. As with any fecal test, a positive result with FIT requires a complete colonic examination with colonoscopy.

Stool DNA test. Detection of altered DNA from exfoliated tumor cells is being investigated as a screening test for colorectal cancer. Screening for a panel of mutations in fecal DNA is more effective than the FOBT in detecting colorectal neoplasia, but the sensitivity of both tests is quite low compared with colonoscopy. The use of the stool DNA test for screening purposes is still an evolving technology but guidelines in North America have already included it as an acceptable option for screening for colorectal cancer. Although the manufacturer of the test kit recommends repeating the exam every 5 years, the ideal interval between tests is not yet known.

Flexible sigmoidoscopy with a 60 cm scope can detect 40–60% of all colorectal cancers and polyps. Several case–control studies have demonstrated that screening by sigmoidoscopy reduces mortality from colorectal cancer by two-thirds for tumors located within the reach of the sigmoidoscope. There is also evidence that flexible sigmoidoscopy reduces the incidence of colorectal cancer in the screened population compared with non-screened controls.

The procedure is fast, requires minimal preparation, and it can be performed in an office-based setting, as conscious sedation is not necessary. The effectiveness of flexible sigmoidoscopy as a screening method requires insertion to at least 40 cm from the anal verge. The presence of adenomatous polyps in the rectosigmoid colon increases the probability of finding additional polyps or cancers in more proximal segments of the large bowel. Thus, if an adenomatous polyp is found during flexible sigmoidoscopy, the patient should undergo a complete colonoscopy. A 5-year interval between studies is considered adequate.

Combined FOBT and flexible sigmoidoscopy. Although the evidence for combining the FOBT and flexible sigmoidoscopy is weak, some studies have shown that the combination of the two screening methods is more effective than each one separately in detecting colorectal neoplasia. The combined approach has the theoretical advantage of detecting lesions located throughout the colon, but its impact on mortality from colorectal cancer is unknown. Annual FOBT combined with flexible sigmoidoscopy every 5 years is a common screening method for the average-risk population in the USA.

Colonoscopy is the most effective procedure for the diagnosis of colorectal polyps and cancers, but its efficacy as a screening test for colorectal cancer has not been tested in a prospective randomized trial. However, there is strong evidence that colonoscopy and polypectomy reduces the incidence of colorectal cancer and associated mortality.

Colonoscopy is more effective than a single FOBT combined with sigmoidoscopy in detecting advanced colonic neoplasia in both men and women. However, colonoscopy is inconvenient, requires dietary modification and bowel preparation, is usually performed under conscious sedation, and carries a risk of complications of 1–2 per 1000. For average-risk individuals colonoscopy screening should start at 50 years of age and should be repeated every 10 years.

Double-contrast barium enema can detect most of the clinically important lesions in the colon but, as with colonoscopy, its effectiveness as a screening test for colorectal cancer is based only on indirect evidence. A double-contrast barium enema every 5 years should provide the same degree of protection as the other screening strategies.

Computed tomography colonography involves thin-section helical CT after standard bowel preparation, followed by three-dimensional reconstruction. CTC identifies 90% of cancers or adenomas measuring more than 10 mm in diameter in asymptomatic individuals 50 years of age or older. It is more sensitive than other screening methods, but can miss flat lesions and polyps smaller than 10 mm in diameter. CTC obviates some of the drawbacks of colonoscopy, such as the need for sedation, but has also downstream consequences: it delivers a dose of radiation that may become substantial with repeated examinations, and detects extracolonic incidental findings that may trigger expensive diagnostic investigations. In addition, patients with lesions found on CTC need a full visualization of the colon by colonoscopy. CTC is now considered an acceptable screening alternative for average-risk individuals, starting at 50 years of age; the optimal interval between examinations is as yet uncertain.

Risk factors

Three-quarters of colorectal cancers occur in people who do not have any particular predisposing factors and who are therefore considered to be at average risk for colorectal cancer. The remaining 25% of patients have risk factors that predispose them to the development of colorectal cancer (Table 4.1).

TABLE 4.1

Risk factors for colorectal cancer

- Family history of colorectal neoplasia
  - carcinoma
  - adenoma (< 60 years of age)
- Past history of colorectal neoplasm
  - carcinoma
  - adenoma
- Inflammatory bowel disease
  - chronic ulcerative colitis
  - Crohn's disease

- Familial adenomatous polyposis (FAP)
  - Gardner's syndrome
  - Turcot's syndrome
  - attenuated polyposis
- MYH-associated polyposis (MAP)
- Hereditary non-polyposis colorectal cancer (HNPCC)
- Juvenile polyposis
- Hamartomas

Family history. First-degree relatives of patients with colorectal cancer or polyps have an increased risk of developing colorectal cancer. The severity of the risk increases with the number of relatives affected and with an early age of cancer diagnosis.

Previous history of colorectal cancer. Patients who have survived a colorectal cancer have four times the lifetime risk of developing a new (metachronous) colorectal cancer than people with average risk.

Inflammatory bowel disease. Patients with ulcerative colitis or Crohn's disease have an increased risk for the development of colorectal cancer compared with the general population. The risk is highest among patients whose inflammatory bowel disease:

- was diagnosed at an early age
- extends proximal to the splenic flexure
- has lasted longer than 8 years.

The colorectal cancers associated with inflammatory bowel disease often do not develop from benign adenomatous polyps but from flat areas of dysplasia, which makes early diagnosis particularly difficult. However, fewer than 1% of all colorectal cancers are associated with inflammatory bowel disease. Screening recommendations for patients with inflammatory bowel disease are given in Table 4.2.

Hamartomas. Patients with hereditary syndromes characterized by the presence of hamartomas in the small and large bowel are at increased risk for the development of colorectal cancer. However, the magnitude of the increase is unknown.

Hereditary colorectal cancer syndromes

Familial adenomatous polyposis (FAP) is an autosomal dominant disease characterized by the development in the teens or early twenties of hundreds or thousands of adenomatous polyps throughout the large bowel (see Chapter 1). If untreated, almost all patients with FAP will develop colorectal cancer by the fourth or fifth decade of life. FAP is responsible for 1% of all colorectal cancers. The disease has several phenotypic variants such as Gardner's syndrome (familial colorectal cancer, osteomas and desmoid tumors), Turcot's syndrome (familial colorectal cancer and brain tumors) and attenuated FAP (fewer than 100 polyps developing later in life). The FAP syndrome is the result of a mutation of the *adenomatous polyposis coli* (*APC*) gene. The location of the mutation within the gene is variable, accounting for the different phenotypic variants of the disease.

MYH-associated polyposis (MAP) is an autosomal recessive predisposition to the formation of polyps and early-onset colorectal cancer. It was first described in 2002 and thus clinical data are still limited. Patients with MAP typically have between 10 and 100 adenomas, but colorectal cancer can occur in the absence of synchronous polyps. Since the condition is inherited recessively, the siblings of an affected person are at 25% risk of having the condition.

Lynch syndrome is characterized by the development of colorectal cancers in several members of the same family, some of them at an early age. The syndrome is caused by germline mutations in the genes coding for mismatch repair (MMR) proteins, which are responsible for the correction of errors that occur during DNA replication. The syndrome often features multiple synchronous cancers, which are frequently located proximal to the splenic flexure. Some patients have an increased incidence of extracolonic malignancies (of the upper gastrointestinal, urinary and female reproductive tracts). In contrast to the polyposis that is pathognomonic for FAP, there is no phenotypic marker for Lynch syndrome.

Lynch syndrome is also called hereditary non-polyposis colorectal cancer (HNPCC). The diagnosis of HNPCC is based on families meeting the Amsterdam clinical criteria rather than on the basis of germline mutations in the MMR genes. It is now recognized that some families fulfill the Amsterdam I and II clinical criteria but the MMR pathway is normal. These families are likely to have cancer because of mutations in other genes or perhaps because of a shared environmental exposure. The term 'familial colorectal cancer syndrome X' is now used for those families who meet the Amsterdam clinical criteria but in whom the MMR genes are intact. The Amsterdam I criteria are:

- the existence of three or more relatives with colorectal cancer, one of whom is a first-degree relative of the other two
- the involvement of at least two consecutive generations
- at least one patient being younger than 50 years of age.

The Amsterdam criteria II include the extracolonic tumors commonly observed in HNPCC, such as cancers of the endometrium, urinary tract and upper gastrointestinal tract.

Screening recommendations

Patients with symptoms of colorectal cancer should undergo the appropriate diagnostic studies; they are not candidates for screening. Screening recommendations for the general population are based on individual risk assessment (see Table 4.2).

Average risk. People at average risk for the development of colorectal cancer (asymptomatic men and women over 50 years of age in the USA and 60 in the UK without risk factors) could undergo yearly FOB testing, combined with flexible sigmoidoscopy every 5 years. People with a positive FOBT or a polyp identified by flexible sigmoidoscopy should have the entire colon and rectum examined by colonoscopy.

TABLE 4.2

Recommendations for screening and surveillance for colorectal cancer

	Risk category	Recommendation
Average risk		
• 65–75% of CRC • Lifetime risk 5%	• Everyone aged 50 years and above without other risk factors (60 in UK)	• FOBT plus flexible sigmoidoscopy or • Total examination of the colon (if requested and implications are understood)*
Moderate risk		
• 20–30% of CRC • Lifetime risk 10–30%	• One first-degree relative with CRC or polyps diagnosed at 60 years of age or older • Two second-degree relatives with CRC	• Screening options at intervals recommended for average-risk individuals
	• One first-degree relative with CRC or polyps diagnosed below 60 years of age or • Two first-degree relatives of any age	• Colonoscopy
High risk		
• 3–5% of CRC • Lifetime risk 50%	• FAP: child or sibling of affected patient	• Sigmoidoscopy • Referral to specialist • Genetic testing
	• HNPCC: at-risk patient whose family fits Amsterdam criteria or positive gene test	• Colonoscopy • Offer genetic testing • Gynecologic screening for women

Age to begin (years)	Interval
• 50	• Annual FOBT • Flexible sigmoidoscopy every 5 years • Colonoscopy every 10 years or • Double-contrast barium enema + flexible sigmoidoscopy every 5 years
• 40	• Same as above until first colonoscopy • Follow-up colonoscopy every 5 years
• 40 or • 10 years before youngest case in family	• Every 5 years for negative examination
• 12, if patient is at risk or carrier • Upper GI endoscopy every 1–2 years after diagnosis • 20–25 years, or 10 years before youngest case in immediate family	• Annually until colectomy (performed if polyps appear) • Every 2 years until 40 years of age, then • Annually

CONTINUED

43

TABLE 4.2 (CONTINUED)

Risk category	Recommendation
Surveillance of people at increased risk	
• Small rectal hyperplastic polyp	• Screening options at intervals recommended for average-risk individuals
• 1 or 2 small tubular adenomas (< 1 cm)	• Colonoscopy
• 3–10 tubular adenomas, large tubular adenomas (> 1 cm), or adenomas with tubulovillous features or high-grade dysplasia	• Colonoscopy
• More than 10 adenomas in one examination	• Colonoscopy
• Previous resection for curative intent of CRC	• Colonoscopy
• Inflammatory bowel disease	• Colonoscopy with surveillance biopsies for dysplasia

*Differs between UK and USA.
CRC, colorectal cancer; FAP, familial adenomatous polyposis; FOBT, fecal occult blood test; GI, gastrointestinal; HNPCC, hereditary non-polyposis colorectal cancer.

Double-contrast barium enema every 5 years or colonoscopy every 10 years are accepted screening alternatives in the average-risk population. CTC every 5 years is also an option. Digital rectal examination should be performed at the time of sigmoidoscopy or colonoscopy in all individuals.

Age to begin (years)	Interval
• 5 years after polypectomy	• 5-year interval for normal examination
• 3 years after clearing the colon	• 5 years if colonoscopy is normal or finds fewer than 3 small polyps
• Less than 3 years after initial polypectomy	• Consider genetic counseling for hereditary syndrome
• A total colon examination should be done at time of resection	• 1 year after resection, then every 3 years if normal, then every 5 years if normal
• 8 years after start of pancolitis	• Every 1–2 years
• 12–15 years after left-sided colitis	• Colectomy is recommended for any dysplasia

Moderate risk. Individuals with a first-degree relative (parent, sibling or child) with colorectal cancer or adenomatous polyps diagnosed before 60 years of age should start screening with colonoscopy at 40 years of age, or 10 years younger than the earliest diagnosis in their family, whichever comes first. The test should be repeated every 5 years. People with one first-degree relative diagnosed with colorectal cancer or adenomatous polyp diagnosed at 60 years of age or older, or with two or more second-degree relatives (grandparent, grandchild, aunt, uncle, niece, nephew, half-sibling) with colorectal cancer or adenomatous polyps at any age, should undergo screening as average-risk individuals but starting at 40 years of age. Patients with one second-degree relative or one or more third-degree relatives (first cousin) affected are considered to be at average risk.

High risk. This category includes individuals from families diagnosed as having hereditary forms of colorectal cancer. At-risk members of families with hereditary cancer syndromes should be informed about the benefits and limitations of genetic counseling and genetic testing.

Familial adenomatous polyposis. Once the diagnosis of FAP is established, the patient should undergo colectomy or a yearly colonoscopy until colectomy. Upper gastrointestinal endoscopy should be performed every 1–2 years. Siblings and children of a patient with FAP should start surveillance by flexible sigmoidoscopy at puberty.

MYH-associated polyposis. Depending on the individual, age of presentation and number and size of polyps, the patient may be advised to undergo a prophylactic colectomy or yearly colonoscopy from 25 years of age. Upper gastrointestinal surveillance should be performed following the guidelines for patients with FAP.

Lynch syndrome. Individuals from families fitting the Amsterdam criteria for HNPCC should have a colonoscopy at 20–25 years of age, every 2 years until 40 years of age, and yearly thereafter. Genetic counseling and testing should be considered.

Surveillance of people at increased risk. Patients undergoing endoscopic excision of a small (< 1 cm) adenomatous polyp (Figure 4.3) should have the entire colon examined at the time of the polypectomy. Colonoscopy should be repeated 5 years later. If the test is negative, they should then follow the screening recommendations for average risk.

Patients with more than three adenomas, adenomas with villous features or high-grade dysplasia, or a large adenomatous polyp (> 1 cm) who have their entire colon examined at the time of polypectomy should

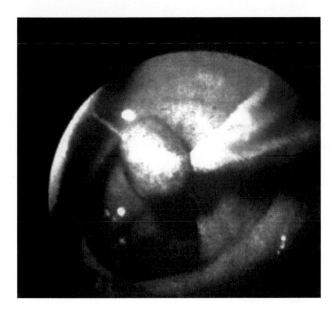

Figure 4.3
Local polypectomy for polyp in sigmoid colon indicated by positive fecal occult blood test.

have their colon examined 3 years later and, if normal, every 5 years thereafter.

A complete colonic examination should be carried out before surgery in any patient undergoing curative resection for colorectal cancer. The colonoscopy should be repeated at 1 year to exclude metachronous lesions. If the examination at 1 year is normal, it should be repeated after 3 years, and every 5 years thereafter if the previous one was normal.

Consequences of screening

The full spectrum of clinical consequences of screening, other than the prevention of deaths from colorectal cancer, is difficult to predict because every screening strategy initiates a cascade of events, each one with uncertain probability. The rate of false-positive tests, the number of colonoscopies performed, the complications of the screening and diagnostic tests, and the number of patients that may require surveillance as a consequence of screening are complex events that happen at different times over several decades. However, cost-effectiveness analysis in the USA has demonstrated that screening for colorectal cancer in average-risk patients according to the strategies

47

suggested above compares favorably with other healthcare interventions such as mammography or treatment of mild hypertension.

A national screening program for people over 60 years old has been initiated in the UK using FOB testing every 2 years.

Implementation of guidelines

The general population has little awareness of the risks of colorectal cancer or its symptoms; the number of individuals participating in screening programs is therefore low. The spread of information to patients is an essential part of the screening program. Primary care providers have the responsibility to inform their patients about their risk of colorectal cancer, the benefits of screening and the different strategies, and to set up a system to implement these guidelines.

Key points – screening and surveillance

- Screening for colorectal cancer and polyps is effective in reducing mortality from colorectal cancer at costs comparable to other cancer screening programs.
- Screening recommendations are based on individual risk as determined by personal and family history.
- Average-risk individuals should start screening at 50 years of age (60 in the UK) with any of the available tests.
- Relatives of patients with colorectal cancer or polyps should be screened regularly by colonoscopy.
- First-degree relatives of patients with familial adenomatous polyposis should have an annual sigmoidoscopy, starting at 10–12 years of age.
- From 20–25 years of age, individuals with Lynch syndrome should have a colonoscopy every 2 years until 40 years of age and annually thereafter.

Key references

Al-Tassan N, Chmiel NH, Maynard J et al. Inherited variants of MYH associated with somatic G:C-->T:A mutations in colorectal tumors. *Nat Genet* 2002;30:227–32.

Frazier AL, Colditz GA, Fuchs CS, Kuntz KM. Cost-effectiveness of screening for colorectal cancer in the general population. *JAMA* 2000;284:1954–61.

Hampel H, Frankel WL, Martin E et al. Screening for the Lynch syndrome (hereditary nonpolyposis colorectal cancer). *N Engl J Med* 2005;352:1851–60.

Imperiale TF, Glowinski EA, Lin-Cooper C et al. Five-year risk of colorectal neoplasia after negative screening colonoscopy. *N Engl J Med* 2008;359:1218–24.

Imperiale TF, Ransohoff DF, Itzkowitz SH et al. Fecal DNA versus fecal occult blood for colorectal-cancer screening in an average-risk population. *N Engl J Med* 2004; 351:2704–14.

Johnson CD, Chen MH, Toledano AY et al. Accuracy of CT colonography for detection of large adenomas and cancers. *N Engl J Med* 2008;359:1207–17.

Kim DH, Pickhardt PJ, Taylor AJ et al. CT colonography versus colonoscopy for the detection of advanced neoplasia. *N Engl J Med* 2007;357:1403–12.

Levin B, Lieberman DA, McFarland B et al. Screening and surveillance for the early detection of colorectal cancer and adenomatous polyps, 2008: a joint guideline from the American Cancer Society, the US Multi-Society Task Force on Colorectal Cancer, and the American College of Radiology. *Gastroenterology* 2008;134: 1570–95.

Lieberman DA, Weiss DG, Bond JH et al. Use of colonoscopy to screen asymptomatic adults for colorectal cancer. *N Engl J Med* 2000;343: 162–8.

Lieberman DA, Weiss DG, Harford WV et al. Five-year colon surveillance after screening colonoscopy. *Gastroenterology* 2007;133:1077–85.

Lieberman DA, Weiss DG, Veterans Affairs Cooperative Study Group 380. One-time screening for colorectal cancer with combined fecal occult-blood testing and examination of the distal colon. *N Engl J Med* 2001;345:555–60.

Pignone M, Saha S, Hoerger T, Mandelblatt J. Cost-effectiveness analyses of colorectal cancer screening: a systematic review for the U.S. Preventive Services Task Force. *Ann Intern Med* 2002;137:96–104.

Regula J, Rupinski M, Kraszewska E et al. Colonoscopy in colorectal-cancer screening for detection of advanced neoplasia. *N Engl J Med* 2006;355:1863–72.

Rex DK, Kahi CJ, Levin B et al. Guidelines for colonoscopy surveillance after cancer resection: a consensus update by the American Cancer Society and the US Multi-Society Task Force on Colorectal Cancer. *Gastroenterology* 2006;130:1865–71.

Sampson JR, Dolwani S, Jones S et al. Autosomal recessive colorectal adenomatous polyposis due to inherited mutations of MYH. *Lancet* 2003;362:39–41.

Schoenfeld P, Cash B, Flood A et al. Colonoscopic screening of average-risk women for colorectal neoplasia. *N Engl J Med* 2005;352:2061–8.

Sieber OM, Lipton L, Crabtree M et al. Multiple colorectal adenomas, classic adenomatous polyposis, and germ-line mutations in MYH. *N Engl J Med* 2003;348:791–9.

Winawer SJ, Zauber AG, Ho MN et al. Prevention of colorectal cancer by colonoscopic polypectomy. *N Engl J Med* 1993;329:1977–81.

Treatment of colorectal cancer is primarily surgical. Treatment of cancers located above or below the peritoneal reflection should be considered separately, as anatomic considerations affect the surgical technique and the use of adjuvant chemotherapy and radiotherapy. However, some aspects, such as diagnostic evaluation and preoperative preparation, apply equally to cancers in both the colon and rectum.

Preoperative preparation

The patient should undergo adequate preoperative evaluation to:

- confirm the diagnosis
- exclude synchronous colorectal cancer or polyps
- determine the local and regional extent of the disease
- exclude the presence of distant metastases
- investigate the patient's overall medical condition, paying particular attention to continence.

The colon harbors the largest number of bacteria, mostly anaerobes, in the gastrointestinal tract. Infection of the surgical site, either superficial or intra-abdominal, secondary to spillage of fecal matter, is a potential complication of colorectal surgery. Reduction of the bacterial load in the colon by mechanical bowel cleansing and oral antibiotics has traditionally been considered an important aspect of the preoperative management of patients undergoing colon or rectal surgery. However, the results of several prospective randomized trials indicate that antegrade mechanical bowel preparation does not reduce the risk of complications, including surgical site infection, after colon surgery. However, a mechanical bowel preparation is often used when intraoperative colonoscopy is required for localized small lesions. The administration of intravenous antibiotics, maintenance of normothermia and administration of supplemental oxygen during surgery have been proven to reduce the risk of surgical site infection in patients undergoing colorectal surgery.

Colon cancer

Surgery. At the time of performing the laparotomy, the entire peritoneal cavity is examined in order to exclude metastatic disease, particularly in the liver, omentum and pelvis. The small bowel is also inspected for any unsuspected pathology. Curative surgical treatment of colon cancer requires resection of the segment of the intestine harboring the tumor, the adjacent mesentery containing the draining lymph nodes, and any organ or tissue adherent to the tumor. Most adhesions between the tumor and adjacent organs are inflammatory, but tumor infiltration cannot be excluded before resection. Infiltration to adjacent organs reduces the likelihood of cure.

The extent of surgical resection depends on the location of the tumor in relation to the major blood vessels (Figure 5.1). The lymphatics draining the bowel run parallel to the mesenteric blood vessels. Enough of the mesentery is resected to obtain at least 12 lymph nodes, the

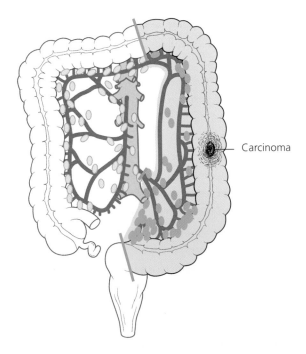

Carcinoma

Figure 5.1 Extent of resection of carcinoma of the descending or sigmoid colon.

minimum number required for accurate staging. If more than one cancer is present in different segments of the colon, or when the cancer is associated with multiple neoplastic polyps, a subtotal colectomy with ileorectal anastomosis may be considered. Intestinal continuity can be re-established in most cases by either a hand-sewn or stapled anastomosis.

Patients found to have metastatic disease at the time of surgery will probably require a palliative resection to prevent obstruction and hemorrhage from the primary tumor. An extensive mesenteric resection is not usually necessary in this situation. Occasionally, a bypass procedure is the only possibility.

Laparoscopic resection of the colon for colorectal cancer is as effective as open surgery in terms of adequate margins and lymph node harvest. However, the suitability of this procedure depends on the expertise available.

After the operation, the bowel is maintained at rest until the ileus resolves. A nasogastric tube is not routinely used in the postoperative period. The most common postoperative complications are:

- incisional wound infection
- atelectasis
- urinary tract infection
- deep venous thrombosis
- anastomotic dehiscence.

Adjuvant chemotherapy. Survival after curative resection for colon cancer is directly related to the pathological stage of the disease.

Stage I or Dukes A disease is associated with a good prognosis, with a 5-year survival greater than 80%. Adjuvant systemic chemotherapy is not appropriate for these individuals.

Stage II or Dukes B disease. Several studies conducted in the USA and Europe have demonstrated no survival advantages for patients with stage II colon cancer treated with chemotherapy in addition to surgery compared with surgery alone. Consequently, postoperative chemotherapy is not routinely recommended for patients with stage II colon cancer. However, patients with stage II cancers that have poor prognostic features, such as perforation, lymphovascular space invasion or involvement of the visceral peritoneum (T4), may be individually considered for adjuvant chemotherapy or, preferably, entered into a clinical trial.

Stage III or Dukes C disease. In patients with lymph node metastases who are undergoing resection alone, the 5-year survival drops to 25–55%, depending on the degree of bowel wall invasion and number of lymph nodes involved. Results from various prospective studies indicate that patients with stage III colon cancer benefit from postoperative adjuvant chemotherapy.

For about 15 years, standard adjuvant chemotherapy involved the administration of fluorouracil and folinic acid (leucovorin), typically by bolus or infusion in a 6-month regimen. Adjuvant treatment can now be administered orally using capecitabine, a prodrug of fluorouracil. Irrespective of the route of administration, the relative improvement in survival using fluorouracil-based chemotherapy is about 33%, which is roughly equivalent to a 10% absolute improvement in survival. Adding oxaliplatin to fluorouracil chemotherapy offers a further improvement in disease-free survival compared with fluorouracil and folinic acid alone. The relative benefit in terms of disease-free survival is about 25% and the overall survival benefit is predicted to be in the order of 20% (relative benefit).

Other agents such as irinotecan that have been shown to be active in the metastatic setting have not yet shown benefit in the adjuvant setting.

Monoclonal antibodies such as bevacizumab and cetuximab, which are approved for use in the metastatic setting, are currently being assessed in clinical trials in the adjuvant setting.

Future adjuvant chemotherapy regimens. There is increasing evidence to suggest that molecular and genetic features of the primary tumor, including the presence of microsatellite instability and retention of heterozygosity, could predict which patients are likely to respond favorably to adjuvant systemic chemotherapy and indeed to which therapy. It is likely that future studies will include such criteria in their protocols.

Rectal cancer

Most rectal cancers are adenocarcinomas and are biologically indistinguishable from colon cancers; they originate from premalignant lesions, penetrate the bowel wall and the lymphatics in the same fashion, and metastasize to the same organs. Treatment is also primarily surgical. Some anatomic and physiological features give the physician more diagnostic possibilities, but complicate the management of patients with rectal cancer. These include:

- extraperitoneal location within the confines of the pelvis
- anatomic relationship to the urogenital system
- dual blood supply from the mesenteric and iliac vessels
- proximity to the anal sphincter mechanism
- complex physiological function of the rectum
- accessibility.

Surgical treatment of rectal cancer requires consideration of the tumor characteristics such as the size, location, depth of invasion, nodal status and differentiation, and patient-related factors, such as comorbid conditions, anorectal functional status and the patient's wishes. Preoperative evaluation should include:

- complete medical history and physical evaluation
- digital rectal examination to determine the functional status of the anal sphincter and the fixity of distal tumors
- proctoscopic examination to assess the size and location of the tumor(s)
- colonoscopy to diagnose any synchronous neoplastic lesions
- abdominal and pelvic CT to determine the extent of perirectal involvement and the presence of liver metastases
- endorectal ultrasonography or MRI to determine penetration of the bowel wall by the tumor, and the presence of perirectal lymph node metastases.

Radical surgery. At diagnosis, most rectal cancers have already spread beyond the rectal wall, by either direct extension or lymphatic spread, and therefore require radical resection. The radical surgical treatment of rectal cancer follows the classic oncological principles of removing the site of the primary tumor and the regional lymph nodes.

The rectum is removed en bloc with the surrounding mesenteric fat harboring the blood vessels and lymphatics, known as the mesorectum. The superior rectal artery is ligated distal to the take-off of the left colic artery. Involvement of the lateral or circumferential resection margin is strongly correlated with the later local recurrence (which generally has a poor prognosis). Most surgeons therefore now advocate complete excision of the mesorectum. The hypogastric nerves are identified and preserved. A margin of at least 1–2 cm of normal rectum distal to the tumor is included to reduce the risk of anastomotic recurrence. As with colon cancer, any adhesion to adjacent organs, such as the uterus, vagina, bladder or small bowel, is resected en bloc with the rectum.

Restoration of intestinal continuity is an important but secondary consideration and is attempted only if a well-perfused tension-free anastomosis can be performed (low anterior resection, Figure 5.2).

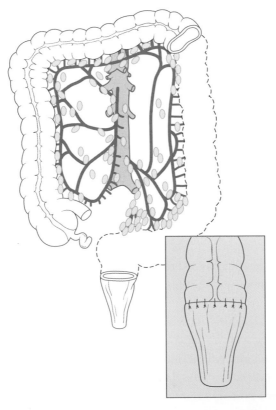

Figure 5.2 Anterior resection for carcinoma of the rectum.

Some surgeons utilize a pouch-anal anastomosis to achieve this with possibly improved function. If the cancer is so low that the 2 cm margin cannot be obtained without compromising the sphincter function, the entire rectum and anus is removed (abdominoperineal resection) and a permanent colostomy is created (Figure 5.3).

Mortality and morbidity. The operative mortality in patients undergoing radical surgery for rectal cancer is low, but morbidity is significant. In addition to the complications common in any patient undergoing major abdominal procedures (atelectasis, wound infection, deep venous thrombosis), these patients are at risk for several specific complications (Table 5.1).

Adjuvant therapy. The treatment paradigm for systemic adjuvant chemotherapy is similar to that used for colon cancer. Unfortunately,

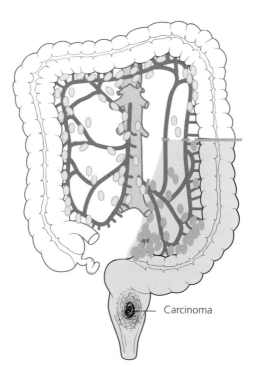

Carcinoma

Figure 5.3 Extent of abdominoperineal resection for carcinoma of the rectum.

TABLE 5.1

Specific complications of surgery for rectal cancer

- Ureteral injury
- Pelvic hemorrhage
- Urinary dysfunction
- Erectile dysfunction (in men)
- Retrograde ejaculation (in men)
- Dyspareunia (in women)
- Anastomotic leak (in patients with low anastomosis)
- Perineal wound infection (in patients undergoing abdominoperineal resection)

patients with rectal cancer have been excluded from many key clinical trials and it therefore remains uncertain whether patients with rectal cancer will benefit from drugs such as oxaliplatin. Many of the studies in rectal cancer have addressed the issue of local recurrence and the impact of preoperative and postoperative radiotherapy on it. Studies that report local recurrence rates are highly variable in terms of quality, and the definition of 'local recurrence' used. As a result, local recurrence rates ranging from 1% to 30% have been reported; such wide variability creates uncertainty about the role of radiotherapy. Adjuvant radiation or chemoradiation administered before or after surgery reduces the rate of local recurrence compared with surgery alone, even in patients treated by total mesorectal excision. There is now conclusive evidence that adjuvant radiation and chemoradiation are more effective and less toxic when administered before rather than after surgery.

In some Scandinavian and European countries radiation is administered in five daily doses of 5 Gy (total dose of 25 Gy) delivered the week before surgery. This regimen has been proven to reduce the rate of local recurrence and, in one trial, to improve survival compared with surgery alone. In other countries, radiation therapy is administered as a long-course regimen: daily doses of 180 cGy, administered 5 days a week for 5–6 weeks (total dose of 5040 cGy) with concomitant continuous infusion of 5-fluorouracil or capecitabine. Surgery is usually performed 6 weeks after finishing the chemoradiation. This long-course regimen may reduce tumor size and stage and is therefore useful for patients with locally advanced tumors.

Patients with ultrasound stage II or stage III rectal cancers have a significant risk of distant metastasis and should also receive systemic adjuvant chemotherapy after recovering from surgery.

Localized disease. A growing number of patients are being diagnosed while their cancer is still localized in the rectal wall. Studies have demonstrated that, in selected patients with tumors localized to the submucosa (T1N0) (Figure 5.4), local excision by either a conventional transanal approach or transanal endoscopic microsurgery results in tumor control equivalent to that of radical surgery, but without the need for a major operation or a permanent colostomy. Local excision as the only form of therapy is not recommended for tumors that penetrate beyond the submucosa. Several studies are investigating the role of chemoradiation followed by local excision for the treatment of rectal cancers that have penetrated into, but not beyond, the muscularis propria of the rectal wall.

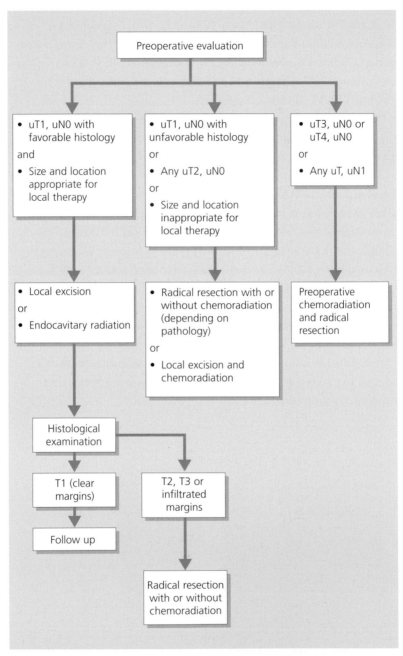

Figure 5.4 Management plan for local therapy of rectal cancer. See
Table 1.2 (pages 16–17) for definitions of TNM staging acronyms.

Key points – treatment of the primary disease

- A preoperative colonoscopy or barium enema is mandatory in any patient with colorectal cancer, in order to exclude synchronous cancers or polyps.
- Surgical resection for colon cancer should be sufficient to ensure negative margins and to provide enough lymph nodes for accurate staging.
- Rectal tumors should be staged using endorectal ultrasonography and/or MRI, in order to select the most appropriate therapy.
- Local excision is adequate for rectal tumors that are limited to the submucosa.
- Radical surgery for rectal cancer requires total mesorectal excision.
- Patients with locally advanced rectal cancer should receive preoperative adjuvant short-course radiation or long-course chemoradiation.
- Patients with colorectal cancer who are at high risk of developing distant metastasis (all stage III, some stage II) should receive postoperative chemotherapy.

Key references

André T, Boni C, Mounedji-Boudiaf L et al. Oxaliplatin, fluorouracil, and leucovorin as adjuvant treatment for colon cancer. *N Engl J Med* 2004; 350:2343–51.

Baxter NN, Garcia-Aguilar J. Organ preservation for rectal cancer. *J Clin Oncol* 2007;25:1014–20.

Brown CJ, Fenech DS, McLeod RS. Reconstructive techniques after rectal resection for rectal cancer. *Cochrane Database Syst Rev* 2008;issue 2: CD006040.

Marr R, Birbeck K, Garvican J et al. The modern abdominoperineal excision: the next challenge after total mesorectal excision. *Ann Surg* 2005;242:74–82.

McArdle CS, McMillan DC, Hole DJ. Impact of anastomotic leakage on long-term survival of patients undergoing curative resection for colorectal cancer. *Br J Surg* 2005; 92:1150–4.

McCormick JT, Gregorcyk SG. Preoperative evaluation of colorectal cancer. *Surg Oncol Clin N Am* 2006;15:39–49.

O'Neil BH, Tepper JE. Current options for the management of rectal cancer. *Curr Treat Options Oncol* 2007;8:331–8.

Peeters KC, Marijnen CA, Nagtegaal ID et al. The TME trial after a median follow-up of 6 years: increased local control but no survival benefit in irradiated patients with resectable rectal carcinoma. *Ann Surg* 2007;246:693–701.

Sauer R, Becker H, Hohenberger W et al. Preoperative versus postoperative chemoradiotherapy for rectal cancer. *N Engl J Med* 2004;351:1731–40.

Swedish Rectal Cancer Trial. Improved survival with preoperative radiotherapy in resectable rectal cancer. *N Engl J Med* 1997;336:980–7.

Wolpin BM, Mayer RJ. Systemic treatment of colorectal cancer. *Gastroenterology* 2008;134:1296–310.

Large bowel obstruction is defined as mechanical blockage to the passage of colonic or rectal contents, with consequent abdominal distension and obstipation. It is a common complication, developing in 7–29% of patients with colorectal cancer. Obstruction is the presenting symptom in up to 15% of patients. Mechanical obstruction should be distinguished from acute colonic pseudo-obstruction, in which colonic and abdominal distension is caused by a functional process for which there is no obvious mechanical cause for the obstruction. This is described in more detail below.

Etiology

Colorectal cancer is responsible for 60–90% of all cases of acute colonic obstruction. Most obstructions occur in the left colon where the feces are solid, the lumen is smaller, and tumors are more likely to be annular. Bowel obstruction secondary to volvulus shows a marked geographic variation: volvulus is rare in the western world, but is responsible for half of all large bowel obstructions in developing countries. Large bowel obstruction secondary to diverticular disease is uncommon, and other causes are extremely rare.

The etiology of acute colonic pseudo-obstruction is unknown, but it is frequently associated with systemic illness, trauma, prolonged immobilization, retroperitoneal pathology, constipating medications, electrolyte imbalance, endocrine disorders and colonic inflammation (Table 6.1).

Pathophysiology

The obstructed bowel undergoes significant changes in motility, secretion and blood flow, which are responsible for the clinical manifestations. Proximal to the obstructed segment, particularly in left-sided obstructions, the colon develops mass action contractions, which cause colic pain. Persistent obstruction and progressive distension lead to colonic hypomotility (Table 6.2).

TABLE 6.1

Etiology of colonic obstruction and clinical conditions predisposing to colonic pseudo-obstruction

Colonic (mechanical) obstruction

- Colorectal cancer
- Diverticulitis
- Volvulus
- Hernia
- Inflammatory bowel disease
- Peritoneal neoplasias
- Radiation stricture
- Anastomotic stricture
- Adhesions
- Foreign bodies
- Fecal impaction

Pseudo-obstruction

- Idiopathic (Ogilvie's syndrome)
- Systemic illness
- Pharmacological agents
  - opioids
  - tranquilizers
  - anticholinergics
  - antidepressants
- Immobility
- Retroperitoneal pathology
- Transplant recipients
- Electrolyte imbalance
- Colonic inflammation
- Endocrine dysfunction (hypothyroidism)

TABLE 6.2

Mechanical aspects of large bowel obstruction

- Increased motility proximal to obstruction
- Emptying of distal bowel
- Distension of proximal bowel
  - increased secretions
  - nitrogen and hydrogen sulfide gas due to bacterial overgrowth
- Bacterial translocation

Colonic obstruction causes progressive abdominal distension as a result of the accumulation of gas (mostly nitrogen from swallowed air), increased fluid secretion and hyperproliferation of anaerobic bacteria. The accumulation of fluid in the distended colon can lead to dehydration.

Progressive distension in the presence of a competent ileocecal valve results in a closed-loop obstruction. The increase in intraluminal pressure can compromise the mucosal blood flow and lead to irreversible ischemia. Tension in the wall of the distended bowel increases in proportion to the fourth power of the radius; the development of ischemia and the risk of subsequent perforation are therefore high, particularly in the cecum, which is the segment of the colon with the largest diameter. The risk of perforation is related not only to the caliber of the colon, but also to the onset of obstruction (higher risk when acute) and the duration of the obstruction.

Mucosal ischemia has been implicated as the cause of a non-specific form of colitis that in some patients develops proximal to the site of obstruction. The presence of ischemia, which can only be diagnosed at the time of surgery, should influence the extent of resection.

Diagnosis

It can be difficult to distinguish acute colonic obstruction from colonic pseudo-obstruction.

Acute colonic obstruction manifests as:
- abdominal discomfort or frank pain (depending on the onset of the obstruction)
- reduction or complete cessation of the passage of flatus and feces
- progressive abdominal distension.

Auscultation of bowel sounds is rarely helpful in the diagnosis of large bowel obstruction. Abdominal tenderness, particularly if associated with fever and leukocytosis, requires immediate evaluation to exclude perforation or ischemia. Obstructing rectal cancers are unusual. Digital rectal examination reveals an empty rectum in most patients with large bowel obstruction.

Colonic pseudo-obstruction can cause symptoms similar to those of acute colonic obstruction. Diagnosis is suggested by:
• the clinical setting (immobilization, opioids, electrolyte imbalance)
• passage of small amounts of gas and feces
• lack of tenderness in a massively distended abdomen.
However, the definitive diagnosis often requires specific radiological tests, such as a water-soluble-contrast enema.

Diagnostic tests
A number of tests are used to aid diagnosis, including:
• radiography
• water-soluble-contrast enema
• colonoscopy
• endoscopy
• abdominal computed tomography (CT) scan.

The plain abdominal film demonstrates colonic distension, with air–fluid levels, and a cut-off at the site of obstruction (Figure 6.1). The absence of small bowel distension indicates a competent ileocecal valve,

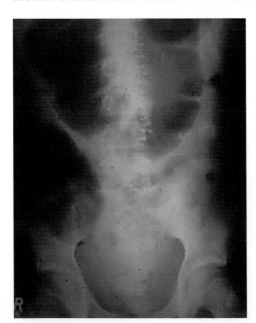

Figure 6.1 Radiograph showing colonic distension.

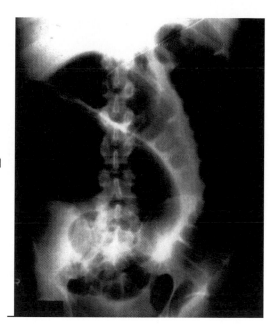

Figure 6.2 Radiograph showing gas in the small bowel.

with an increased risk of cecal perforation. The presence of gas in the small bowel and rectum raises the possibility of ileus or colonic pseudo-obstruction, but radiological findings can be misleading (Figure 6.2). The presence of intramural gas indicates advanced ischemia. A chest radiograph should always be obtained to exclude the presence of pneumoperitoneum.

Water-soluble-contrast enema. This test helps to determine the degree and level of obstruction (Figure 6.3). The flow of contrast to the cecum and the absence of mucosal abnormalities suggests colonic pseudo-obstruction. The osmotic effect of the water-soluble contrast material may have a therapeutic effect in decompressing the colon in these patients. The mucosal detail at the site of obstruction may help to define the cause of the obstruction.

Colonoscopy is a better alternative to contrast enema when confirming the presence of cancer. It may be therapeutic in cases of obstruction secondary to volvulus.

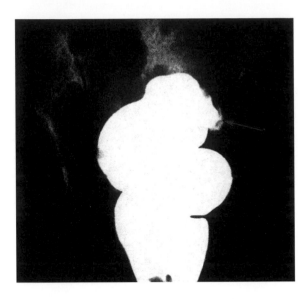

Figure 6.3
Gastrografin enema demonstrating obstruction of the rectosigmoid junction (arrowed).

Abdominal computed tomography locates the transition point between the distended bowel above the obstruction and the collapsed bowel distal to the obstruction. It also provides useful information to differentiate between a malignant obstruction and a colonic obstruction caused by volvulus or diverticulitis. A CT pneumocolon can demonstrate the site and cause of obstruction and provide information about the extent of malignant spread.

Treatment

Patients presenting with obstructing colorectal cancer have higher operative mortality and morbidity and a poorer long-term prognosis than patients undergoing elective resection. Perioperative morbidity and mortality are three times higher with surgery performed for obstruction compared with elective surgery. Cardiopulmonary complications and abdominal sepsis are the major causes of in-hospital mortality and morbidity. The aim in surgery is therefore to minimize morbidity whilst obtaining functional results similar to those obtained in patients undergoing elective resection.

In the absence of perforation, the main differences between patients with obstruction and those with non-obstructing lesions are:

- the pathophysiological consequences of obstruction (dehydration, respiratory compromise, ischemic colitis)
- the fecal load proximal to the point of obstruction
- technical difficulties imposed by a massively distended bowel.

The surgical approach aims to correct these factors.

Preoperative fluid resuscitation and correction of electrolyte imbalances are important in patients with large bowel obstruction. A urinary catheter facilitates fluid management. Unstable patients should be monitored appropriately in the intensive care unit. A nasogastric tube prevents accumulation of swallowed air. Antibiotic prophylaxis with a second-generation cephalosporin or a combination of an aminoglycoside and metronidazole should be given at the time of surgery.

Surgical management depends on the location of the obstruction. Lesions proximal to the splenic flexure are commonly treated by an extended right hemicolectomy with primary anastomosis between the terminal ileum and the non-obstructed colon distal to the lesion. This has the advantage of being a single procedure, removing the entire segment of distended and potentially ischemic bowel, and eliminating the risk of leaving a synchronous tumor in the obstructed colon. Some of these patients develop mild diarrhea but this is usually temporary.

The management of a lesion located distal to the splenic flexure is more controversial (Table 6.3). The three-stage procedure used in the past is rarely used today. A popular choice used to be a two-stage process involving resection of the segment containing the tumor, closure of the rectal stump as a Hartmann's pouch, and construction of an end colostomy, followed by bowel anastomosis at a later date. However, the cumulative mortality and morbidity of both procedures is significant, and at least 30% of patients are left with a permanent colostomy. In most tertiary centers this operation is now limited to situations in which a primary anastomosis is contraindicated (e.g. in the presence of fecal peritonitis from an obstructed and perforated tumor). However, the Hartmann's procedure should be considered for septic or unstable patients, and whenever the quality of the tissues in the pelvis precludes a safe anastomosis.

TABLE 6.3

Surgical alternatives in the treatment of malignant left colon obstruction

Emergency surgery

Three-stage procedure (very rarely necessary)

- Diverting colostomy
- Resection and anastomosis
- Closure of colostomy

Two-stage procedure

- Primary resection, end-colostomy and Hartmann's pouch
- Colorectal anastomosis

One-stage procedures

- Subtotal colectomy and ileorectal anastomosis

or

- Segmental colectomy, intraoperative colon lavage, primary anastomosis

Non-surgical decompression and elective surgery

- YAG laser

or

- Intraluminal stent

The goal today is to relieve the obstruction and treat the cancer in a single operative procedure. Options include:

- treating the obstruction preoperatively (described below), and then preparing the colon for an elective procedure
- subtotal colectomy and ileorectal anastomosis
- segmental resection, intraoperative lavage of the obstructed segment, followed by primary anastomosis.

Non-operative colonic decompression. The obstruction can be relieved preoperatively by either endoluminal resection of the tumor with the help of a YAG laser, or by placement of an expandable endoluminal prosthesis (Figure 6.4). Both procedures relieve the

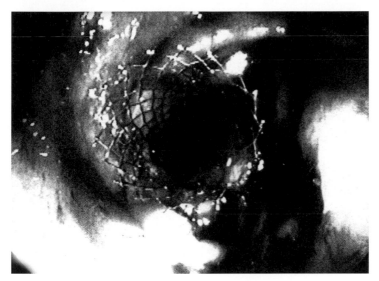

Figure 6.4 An expandable endoluminal prosthesis.

obstruction, allowing non-operative decompression and mechanical preparation of the colon. This enables elective resection to be performed during the same admission. Although no comparative studies of these techniques have been performed, the placement of an endoluminal prosthesis is technically simple and is available in most hospitals. These techniques are contraindicated when there are signs of perforation or colonic ischemia.

Subtotal colectomy with ileorectal anastomosis is a quick operation in which non-distended bowel is used for the anastomosis. This procedure reduces the risk of leaving behind a synchronous tumor in the obstructed portion of the colon, minimizes the risk of fecal spillage, and facilitates follow-up of these patients who have less colon to examine. The disadvantages, however, are a higher incidence of bowel obstruction after ileorectal anastomosis and the development of diarrhea, which may become incapacitating in elderly patients.

Segmental resection with intraoperative colonic lavage and primary anastomosis is a smaller operation and avoids the risk of diarrhea. Disadvantages are the risk of fecal spillage, the use of distended colon for the anastomosis, and the possibility of leaving a synchronous tumor in the obstructed segment of the colon.

Although surgical tradition has condemned the performance of an anastomosis in an unprepared colon, experience accumulated from the management of patients with civilian colon trauma has demonstrated that, under specific circumstances, a primary anastomosis can be performed safely in an unprepared colon provided the bowel looks healthy and there is not extensive soiling in the peritoneal cavity This experience has been transferred to malignant colonic obstruction.

Key points – large bowel obstruction

- Colorectal cancer is the most common cause of colonic obstruction.
- A mechanical obstruction must be distinguished from colonic pseudo-obstruction.
- Patients with colonic obstruction require fluid resuscitation and correction of electrolyte imbalances.
- A complete colonic obstruction is a surgical emergency in order to avoid colonic perforation and peritonitis.
- The goals of surgery are to relieve the obstruction and treat its cause in a single operative procedure.

Key references

Baron TH. Acute colonic obstruction. *Gastrointest Endosc Clin N Am* 2007;17:323–39.

Batke M, Cappell MS. Adynamic ileus and acute colonic pseudo-obstruction. *Med Clin North Am* 2008;92:649–70.

Breitenstein S, Rickenbacher A, Berdajs D et al. Systematic evaluation of surgical strategies for acute malignant left-sided colonic obstruction. *Br J Surg* 2007;94:1451–60.

McArdle CS, Hole DJ. Emergency presentation of colorectal cancer is associated with poor 5-year survival. *Br J Surg* 2004;91:605–9.

The SCOTIA Study Group. Single-stage treatment for malignant left-sided colonic obstruction: a prospective randomized clinical trial comparing subtotal colectomy with segmental resection following intraoperative irrigation. *Br J Surg* 1995;82:1622–7.

Tekkis PP, Kinsman R, Thompson MR et al. The Association of Coloproctology of Great Britain and Ireland study of large bowel obstruction caused by colorectal cancer. *Ann Surg* 2004;240:76–81.

Tilney HS, Lovegrove RE, Purkayastha S et al. Comparison of colonic stenting and open surgery for malignant large bowel obstruction. *Surg Endosc* 2007;21:225–33.

Trompetas V. Emergency management of malignant acute left-sided colonic obstruction. *Ann R Coll Surg Engl* 2008;90:181–6.

Recurrence

Approximately half of patients who undergo surgery for colorectal cancer will develop a recurrence, the majority within 3 years of initial resection.

The pattern of recurrence for colorectal cancer is fairly standard. Patients present with:

- liver metastases
- lung metastases
- a combination of local recurrence and liver metastases
- peritoneal recurrence
- local recurrence
- widespread distant metastases (although this is rare).

A small percentage of patients will present with potentially surgically resectable metastatic disease. For those individuals who undergo a successful resection of metastatic disease, the survival rate at 5 years is approximately 25%. Unfortunately most patients do not have resectable disease, in which case the purpose of treatment is palliative. Palliative care is usually undertaken by a multidisciplinary team that includes medical oncologists, palliative care specialists, general practitioners, stoma nurses, nursing coordinators and counselors. Their role is described in more detail in Chapter 8.

Liver metastases

The liver is the major site of metastases in most individuals (Figure 7.1). Investigation of patients with colorectal liver metastases should determine whether the metastatic disease is resectable. In approximately 10% of patients the metastases are confined to a single lobe, in which case surgery should be considered. Surgery for resection may involve either a segmentectomy or hemi-hepatectomy (Figure 7.2). These procedures are associated with an operative mortality of less than 5%. Three-year survival following resection is approximately 60%; 5-year survival is approximately 25%.

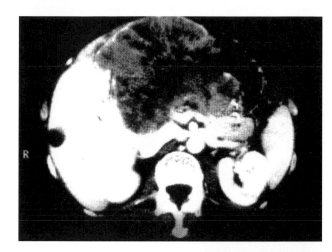

Figure 7.1 Computed tomography scan showing extensive metastasis involving the left lobe and part of the right lobe of the liver.

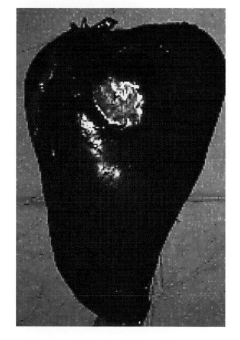

Figure 7.2 Resection specimen following right hemi-hepatectomy for localized liver metastasis.

Before considering resection it is important to ensure that disease is confined to the liver (Table 7.1).

The following therapeutic modalities should be considered in patients with multiple liver metastases for which resection is not appropriate.

TABLE 7.1

Selection criteria for resection of liver metastases

- Preferably confined to single lobe
- No extrahepatic metastases
- Patient fit for major surgery
- No jaundice
- Good liver function
- No local recurrence

Systemic chemotherapy. A combination of fluorouracil and folinic acid (leucovorin), given as an infusion, together with either oxaliplatin or irinotecan is the most effective first-line chemotherapy for metastatic disease. The response rate is approximately 48%, and median survival is about 16 months. This compares with a median survival of about 14 months and a response rate of 20% when using fluorouracil alone.

Oxaliplatin and irinotecan seem to be equally effective partners for fluorouracil when used in the metastatic setting. Expectedly, the use of oxaliplatin or irinotecan is associated with more side effects than using fluorouracil as a single agent. In particular, these agents increase the incidence of gastrointestinal side effects such as diarrhea and nausea, and also neutropenia. Oxaliplatin is associated with peripheral neuropathy, which typically limits the number of treatment cycles to nine.

Rarely, first-line administration of chemotherapy will down-stage liver metastases and may therefore make surgical resection possible. The exact benefit of this approach, if any, is still under investigation, however.

Studies have recently shown that the response to first-line chemotherapy can be further increased by concomitant use of a monoclonal antibody (bevacizumab) that targets circulating vascular endothelial growth factor (VEGF). In these studies, the median survival was between 18 and 20 months when comparing chemotherapy and bevacizumab with chemotherapy alone. The addition of bevacizumab is generally not associated with severe acute toxicities.

Following the failure of first-line treatment, some patients have the option of second- or even third-line chemotherapy. The most effective second-line treatments usually involve the use of a chemotherapy drug such as irinotecan together with a biological therapy, usually an antibody treatment.

The most commonly used antibodies in this setting are those that target the epidermal growth factor receptor pathway on the surface of cancer cells (e.g. cetuximab). The combination of cetuximab and irinotecan doubles the response rate from about 10% to 20% compared with irinotecan alone. Like all biological therapies, cetuximab is very expensive and hence unaffordable by most countries with a national health scheme. Recent data, however, suggest that only those tumors without mutations in the K-*ras* gene may be particularly sensitive to cetuximab (response rates 40%). Molecular testing of colorectal cancers may thus provide an opportunity to preselect those patients in whom cetuximab may be beneficial.

Locoregional chemotherapy. Liver metastases obtain the majority of their blood supply from the hepatic artery. Numerous studies in the past 20 years have used locoregional hepatic arterial chemotherapy to deliver higher and more effective doses of chemotherapy directly to liver metastases. This procedure involves insertion of an arterial catheter into the hepatic artery via the gastroduodenal artery (Figure 7.3). High-dose infusional fluorouracil and fluorourodeoxyuridine (FUDR) can be administered in this way.

Meta-analysis of studies using locoregional chemotherapy has demonstrated an overall improvement in survival compared with systemic chemotherapy, although a recent trial did not find any significant benefit in overall survival between a combination of intrahepatic arterial fluorouracil chemotherapy and systemic folinic acid. Given the morbidity associated with the insertion of implantable intrahepatic devices, however, this technique cannot be recommended outside of a clinical trial setting.

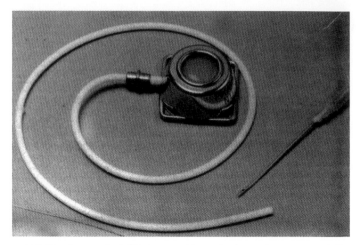

Figure 7.3 The Port-a-Cath® is inserted into the hepatic artery to deliver locoregional chemotherapy to the liver. Photograph courtesy of Deltec, Inc., St Paul, MN, USA.

Interstitial treatment. In selected patients liver tumors can be destroyed in situ by:

- selective internal radiation therapy (SIRT)
- cryotherapy
- interstitial laser photocoagulation
- radiofrequency ablation
- local injection of alcohol.

Each of these techniques has its advocates. There have been reports of improvements in survival following selective interstitial therapy, but it is important to select patients carefully and to realize that current evidence shows these techniques to be purely palliative. Nevertheless, there is increasing enthusiasm for radiofrequency ablation of liver metastases combined with systemic chemotherapy or in association with liver resection – major liver metastases can be resected and smaller anatomically distant ones in the liver can be dealt with by radiofrequency ablation.

Treatment of locally recurrent colon and rectal cancer

Pelvic recurrence is a rare but devastating problem that can occur in patients who have undergone 'curative' resection for rectal cancer. It carries a very poor prognosis, median survival being only 13 months. Uncontrolled pelvic recurrence can be the source of significant disability, pain and tenesmus, and the patient is likely to be distressed by the presence and smell of a necrotic tumor protruding through the perineum.

The incidence of isolated local recurrence is reported to be 3–32%. This variation between series is due not only to factors that affect the risk of local recurrence, but also to differences in the length of follow-up and diagnostic criteria.

Recurrent rectal cancer is difficult to treat; prevention is therefore the key goal of initial treatment. The increasing use of total mesorectal excision (see pages 55–6) is likely to reduce the incidence of major recurrent disease. Isolated pelvic recurrences can be removed surgically provided they do not involve the lateral pelvic sidewall or the upper portion of the sacrum (S2 or above). However, these are complex procedures that should be only attempted in specialized institutions.

Surgery. Autopsy series report that 25–50% of patients with local recurrence have cancer confined to the pelvis when they die; aggressive treatment in these patients therefore seems justified. The extent of surgery depends on:
- the primary operation
- prior use of adjuvant therapy
- the size and location of the recurrence.

Surgery often involves resection of adjacent pelvic organs such as the uterus, vagina, bladder and ureter, the sacrum and bony structures of the pelvic wall; extensive reconstructive surgery is often required. Contraindications for resective surgery include the presence of distant metastases, extensive involvement of the pelvic wall, iliac–venous obstruction and bilateral sciatic pain.

Intraoperative radiotherapy combined with aggressive surgery may improve tumor control and survival in patients who undergo palliative or curative surgical resection for locally recurrent rectal cancer.

Occasionally, recurrence can result in fistulas to the bladder (colovesical fistulas), vagina (colovaginal fistulas) or the abdominal wall. These are serious problems and patients may require palliative surgery, such as colostomy.

An aggressive surgical approach is also warranted for the few patients who develop an isolated local recurrence after surgical treatment of colon cancer. Long-term survival or sustained palliation can be achieved with surgical resection of local recurrences that do not involve vital structures.

Multimodal therapy. Some groups have developed a combined protocol to treat previously non-irradiated biopsy-proven recurrent rectal cancer. The protocol includes preoperative chemoradiation, aggressive surgical resection and selective intraoperative radiation. Preoperative chemoradiation improves resectability and local control.

Radiation therapy is an important therapeutic modality in the management of symptomatic non-resectable recurrent disease. Some series report up to 90% initial pain control and improved quality of life, but no impact on median survival. Radiation therapy, usually combined with chemotherapy, is reserved for patients with non-resectable isolated recurrences.

Other palliative procedures such as stents for ureteral obstruction, colostomy for rectal obstruction in patients with pelvic recurrence, and nerve block may offer significant palliation in selected patients.

Peritoneal metastases

It is not uncommon for patients to develop malignant ascites as a result of multiple peritoneal metastases following surgery for colorectal cancer. This form of recurrence is fatal and there are few treatments to assist. Paracentesis is indicated if the ascites is major and is causing distressing symptoms. This may need to be repeated and can be accompanied by intraperitoneal instillation of chemotherapeutic agents.

Other distant metastases

It is less common for patients with colorectal cancer to develop metastases outside the peritoneal cavity. When such metastases do occur, the most common sites are the lung, brain and bone. Lung or brain metastases that occur as solitary sites of metastases can often be resected; preoperative workup for such cases mirrors that described above for liver metastases. In the past, bone metastases were rare; however, their incidence has increased concomitantly with the improvements in median survival of patients with metastatic cancer. Patients rarely develop metastases outside the peritoneal cavity without the presence of existing liver metastases. It appears that metastases spread from metastases.

Key points – advanced and recurrent disease

- Patients should be carefully assessed before resection of colorectal metastases.
- In patients with resectable metastatic disease the 5-year survival rate is 25%.
- Surgery is not appropriate for most patients with metastatic disease; combination chemotherapy with or without biological therapy is the mainstay of treatment.
- Median survival with state-of-the-art combination therapy is about 20 months.
- Biological therapies are expensive and are not affordable in most countries.

Key references

Bakx R, Visser O, Josso J et al. Management of recurrent rectal cancer: a population based study in greater Amsterdam. *World J Gastroenterol* 2008;14:6018–23.

Kemeny N. Presurgical chemotherapy in patients being considered for liver resection. *Oncologist* 2007;12:825–39.

Miller G, Biernacki P, Kemeny NE et al. Outcomes after resection of synchronous or metachronous hepatic and pulmonary colorectal metastases. *J Am Coll Surg* 2007;205:231–8.

Pawlik TM, Choti MA. Surgical therapy for colorectal metastases to the liver. *J Gastrointest Surg* 2007;11:1057–77.

Pfannschmidt J, Dienemann H, Hoffmann H. Surgical resection of pulmonary metastases from colorectal cancer: a systematic review of published series. *Ann Thorac Surg* 2007;84:324–38.

Wolpin BM, Mayer RJ. Systemic treatment of colorectal cancer. *Gastroenterology* 2008;134: 1296–310.

Multidisciplinary management

Multidisciplinary management is now the established practice for optimal care. For years, surgery has been the mainstay of treatment for patients with colorectal cancer. Once the diagnosis was made, the surgeon was the main – and often the sole – health professional responsible for care of the patient. However, advances in molecular biology, surgical techniques, radiation therapy, chemotherapy, interventional radiology and patient support services have resulted in new treatment options and improved clinical outcomes. Nowadays, the treatment of patients with colorectal cancer frequently requires coordinated decision making by several specialists from different disciplines including nurse specialists, stoma care assistants and a palliative care team. The need for a multidisciplinary approach to the care of a patient with colorectal cancer is particularly evident in some specific clinical scenarios, described below.

Hereditary risk assessment

Identification of some of the genetic mutations responsible for the hereditary colorectal cancer syndromes – familial adenomatous polyposis (FAP), Lynch syndrome and MYH-associated polyposis – has raised the possibility of integrating genetic testing into clinical practice. Many professional societies have now developed guidelines to help clinicians provide genetic counseling and genetic testing for patients who may have a hereditary colorectal cancer syndrome. The results of such counseling and testing may then be used as the basis for recommendations regarding not only the treatment and surveillance of the index patients, but also the screening and counseling of their extended families. Examples of questions that are best addressed by a multidisciplinary team, including the primary care physician, genetic counselor, gastroenterologist and colorectal surgeon, include:

- the extent of a colectomy required in a patient with Lynch syndrome and colorectal cancer

- the choice between prophylactic colectomy or colonoscopy surveillance in an asymptomatic patient with Lynch syndrome (see Chapter 1)
- the timing of colectomy in a patient with attenuated FAP.

A hereditary predisposition to colorectal cancer, although less evident than in patients with FAP, Lynch syndrome or MYH-associated polyposis, is also important in the 25% of patients with a family history of colorectal cancer who do not have germline mutations in the known cancer predisposition genes. Close collaboration between the primary care physician, gastroenterologist and colorectal surgeon is often required to ensure proper surveillance and appropriate screening recommendations for such patients and their families.

Treatment of primary disease

The combination of fluorouracil and folinic acid (leucovorin), together with oxaliplatin, increases the survival of patients with stage III colon cancer compared with surgery alone. The use of combination chemotherapy regimens in the adjuvant setting poses new challenges that require close interaction between medical oncologist and surgeon. Specific issues include:

- the process used to select patients for chemotherapy
- timing of ileostomy closure
- the role of surgery in the management of uncommon side effects of combination chemotherapy such as small bowel injury syndrome.

The care of patients with rectal cancer is based on preoperative tumor staging and histological results. In recent years, patients with stage I rectal cancer have been treated with local excision with (T2N0) or without (T1N0) postoperative chemoradiation. For patients with stage II or stage III rectal cancer, chemoradiation before or after surgery reduces the rate of local recurrence and possibly improves survival compared with surgery alone. Thus, the radiation oncologist has become a key member of the multidisciplinary team.

The need for a multidisciplinary approach is particularly evident in the treatment of patients with stage IV disease. Their treatment must be planned individually, taking into consideration the disease-related symptoms, the patient's overall medical condition, the potential consequences of progression of the primary lesion, and the extent and resectability of the metastatic disease. The selection and timing of the different treatment options – whether surgery, chemotherapy, radiation therapy or any combination of these – must involve the colorectal surgeon, medical oncologist, radiation oncologist, hepatobiliary surgeon and thoracic surgeon. The contributions of additional health professionals from different specialties will be required according to the clinical presentation of individual patients (Figure 8.1).

Treatment of advanced disease

Metastatic disease can rarely be addressed by a single specialist. A hepatobiliary surgeon may resect an isolated liver metastasis, or a thoracic surgeon a lung metastasis, but most patients with metastatic

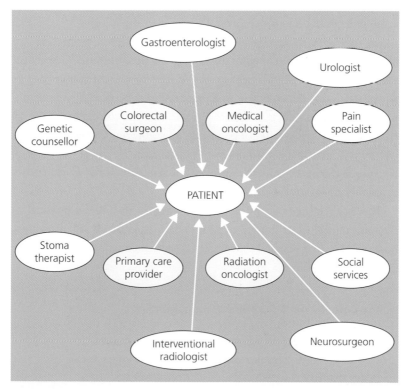

Figure 8.1 A representation of the patient-centered multidisciplinary team in the management of colorectal cancer.

disease usually require several forms of therapy involving more than one specialty. For example, a patient with multiple liver metastases may need systemic chemotherapy, hepatic artery infusional chemotherapy, radiofrequency ablation, or even surgery.

Fortunately, isolated pelvic recurrences after curative-intent surgery for rectal cancer are rare. The role of radical surgery, even in patients with potentially resectable recurrent tumors, remains controversial. However, whether treated with curative-intent surgery or palliative methods, patients with pelvic recurrences require a multidisciplinary approach that involves palliative care and counseling support. In addition to surgery, most of these patients will need preoperative and/or intraoperative radiation and systemic chemotherapy. Curative-intent surgery often demands pelvic exenteration with sacrectomy; the surgical team will therefore include a urologist, a neurosurgeon and a plastic surgeon in addition to the colorectal surgeon.

Patients being treated palliatively often develop bowel or ureteral obstruction, which may require input from an interventional radiologist for placement of a stent or nephrostomy catheter. The contribution of a pain specialist to the treatment of a patient with advanced disease is of inestimable value.

A significant proportion of patients with colorectal cancer need a temporary or permanent stoma. For these patients the contribution of the stomal therapist spans aspects from the selection of the stoma site to the management of stoma complications.

The global effects of the disease and its treatment result in physical distress, physiological stress, financial burden and overall impairment in quality of life that demand the input of a sophisticated patient support system.

Key points – multidisciplinary management

- Early multidisciplinary team consultation is important.
- A single health professional is required to coordinate and summarize the recommendations from the team.

Key references

Cervantes A, Roselló S, Rodríguez-Braun E et al. Progress in the multidisciplinary treatment of gastrointestinal cancer and the impact on clinical practice: perioperative management of rectal cancer. *Ann Oncol* 2008;19(Suppl 7):vii266–72.

Minsky BD. Multidisciplinary case teams: an approach to the future management of advanced colorectal cancer. *Br J Cancer* 1998;77 (Suppl 2):1–4.

Nicholls RJ, Tekkis PP. Multidisciplinary treatment of cancer of the rectum: a European approach. *Surg Oncol Clin N Am* 2008; 17:533–51,viii.

Rougier P, Neoptolemos JP. The need for a multidisciplinary approach in the treatment of advanced colorectal cancer: a critical review from a medical oncologist and surgeon. *Eur J Surg Oncol* 1997;23:385–96.

Progress in our understanding of the biology, natural history, prevention and treatment of colorectal cancer during the past decade has resulted in a persistent decline in mortality from this disease. The future prospects for different areas related to this disease will probably help to accelerate this trend in coming years.

Biology

Over the last few years our knowledge about the genetic and molecular alterations that underlie the development and progression of colorectal cancer have been refined. It is now recognized that epigenetic changes in cancer cells outnumber genetic alterations by 40 to 1. The epigenetic changes control the expression of genes without affecting the DNA sequence. Most microsatellite unstable colorectal cancers occur because of an epigenetic change (methylation) in the *hMLH1* gene. This change completely silences this gene. In contrast to genetic changes, epigenetic alterations are potentially reversible, offering the possibility of developing new therapies. Recently it has also been shown that some patients are born with epigenetic alterations in key genes and as a consequence they are predisposed to developing colorectal cancer.

The genetic make-up of tumor cells is also being used to identify patients who are most likely to respond to therapy. Given the price of new targeted cancer therapies, the careful selection of patients has never been more imperative.

Prevention

The genetic basis of a familial predisposition to colorectal tumors has become more evident in recent years, but there is a large body of evidence supporting the influence of several environmental factors in the development of colorectal cancer. Changes in some of these factors, such as decreasing intake of fat and increasing intake of dietary fiber, and the use of calcium and vitamin C supplements, may reduce the incidence of colorectal cancer. There is increasing evidence that non-steroidal anti-inflammatory drugs (NSAIDs) have a protective effect. Studies with gene-knockout mice suggest that inhibition of the cyclooxygenase type 2 pathway by NSAIDs may be important.

Screening

Although the fecal occult blood test (FOBT) has low sensitivity, poor specificity and poor predictive value, its use as a screening tool has nevertheless been shown to reduce mortality from colorectal cancer. Additional screening with flexible sigmoidoscopy is likely to have further benefits. We need to identify groups most at risk so that screening is as cost-effective as possible. In the future, improved screening tools are likely to replace the FOBT. However many countries including the UK have national screening programs.

Diagnosis

Virtual colonoscopy (computer tomography colonography), the relatively new method of colonic examination involving spiral computed tomography and virtual-reality computer technology, may have a significant impact on the acceptance and safety of colorectal cancer screening and diagnosis. Other diagnostic modalities, such as positron emission tomography, PET/CT and magnetic resonance imaging, are of increasing importance in the diagnosis and staging of colorectal cancer.

Useful addresses

UK

BASO – The Association for Cancer Surgery
at The Royal College of Surgeons
35–43 Lincoln's Inn Fields
London WC2A 3PE
Tel: +44 (0)20 7405 5612
admin@baso.org.uk
www.baso.org.uk

Association of Coloproctology of Great Britain and Ireland
at The Royal College of Surgeons of England (address as above)
Tel: +44 (0)20 7973 0307
acpgbi@asgbi.org.uk
www.acpgbi.org.uk

Beating Bowel Cancer
Harlequin House, 7 High Street
Teddington TW11 8EE
Tel: 08450 719300
Nurse advice service: 08450 719301
nurse@beatingbowelcancer.org
www.beatingbowelcancer.org

Bowel Cancer UK
7 Rickett Street, London SW6 1RU
Tel: +44 (0)20 7381 9711
admin@bowelcanceruk.org.uk
Tel: +44 (0)131 225 5333
scotadmin@bowelcanceruk.org.uk
www.bowelcanceruk.org.uk

Cancer Research UK
PO Box 123, Lincoln's Inn Fields
London WC2A 3PX
Tel: +44 (0)20 7242 0200
Tel (support): +44 (0)20 7121 6699
www.cancerresearchuk.org

Colorectal surgeon
www.colorectalsurgeon.org.uk
Includes links to resources for colorectal surgeons.

Colostomy Association
2 London Court, East Street
Reading RG1 4QL
Tel: +44 (0)118 939 1537
Helpline: 0800 328 4257
cass@colostomyassociation.org.uk
www.colostomyassociation.org.uk

Ileostomy and Internal Pouch Support Group
Peverill House, 1–5 Mill Road
Ballyclare, Co. Antrim BT39 9DR
Tel: +44 (0)28 9334 4043
Helpline: 0800 0184 724
info@iasupport.org
www.iasupport.org.uk

Macmillan Cancer Support
89 Albert Embankment
London SE1 7UQ
Tel: +44 (0)20 7840 7841
Helpline: 0808 808 00 00
www.macmillan.org.uk

National Association for Colitis
and Crohn's Disease
4 Beaumont House, Sutton Road
St Albans, Herts AL1 5HH
Tel: 0845 130 2233
Support line: 0845 130 3344
info@nacc.org.uk
www.nacc.org.uk

NHS Bowel Cancer Screening
Programme
Tel: 0800 707 6060
www.cancerscreening.nhs.uk/bowel

USA
American Cancer Society
www.cancer.org.

American Society of Colon and
Rectal Surgeons
85 W. Algonquin Road, Suite 550
Arlington Heights, IL 60005
Tel: +1 847 290 9184
ascrs@fascrs.org
www.fascrs.org

MD Anderson Cancer Center
University of Texas
www3.mdanderson.org/depts/hcc

National Cancer Institute
US National Institutes of Health
www.cancer.gov

National Comprehensive Cancer
Network
www.nccn.org

STOP Colon/Rectal Cancer
Foundation
www.coloncancerprevention.org

International
Cancer Institute NSW (Australia)
PO Box 41, Alexandria NSW 1435
Tel: +61 (0)2 8374 5600
information@cancerinstitute.org.au
www.cancerinstitute.org.au
eviQ Cancer Treatments Online:
www.eviq.org.au

Colorectal Cancer Association of
Canada
Tel (Montreal): +1 514 875 7745
Tel (Toronto): +1 416 920 4333
Toll-free: 1 877 50 26566
information@colorectal-cancer.ca
www.colorectal-cancer.org.ca

Colorectal Surgical Society of
Australia & New Zealand
PO Box 725, Camberwell South LPO
VIC 3124, Australia
Tel: +61 (0)3 9889 9458
secretariat@cssanz.org
www.cssa.org.au

Index

What the reviewers say:

...the sort of publication that anyone willing to take the time to study the condition of epilepsy will gain enormous benefit from. It packs a load of information into just 138 pages and is, at this point in time, easily the most up-to-date book on current antiepileptic drugs

Mike Glynn, President, International Bureau for Epilepsy
on *Fast Facts – Epilepsy*, revised 4th edn, Jan 2010

Brilliant

Dr David Sanders, Chair, BSG Small Bowel and Nutrition Committee
on *Fast Facts – Celiac Disease*, 2nd edn, Sep 2009

The main strengths of the book are the combination of attractive figures and schemes with simple but clear messages in the text...this attractive small book is very useful for general practitioners, non-rheumatologists and allied health professionals

on *Fast Facts – Osteoarthritis*
Rheumatology, Sep 2009

An outstanding up-to-date compilation of facts on psoriasis, a must-read for any healthcare provider with an interest in psoriasis, whether casual or in-depth

Dr Gerald Krueger, Professor of Dermatology, University of Utah School of Medicine,
on *Fast Facts – Psoriasis*, 2nd edn, Jan 2009

This concise, up-to-date, well-illustrated text represents excellent value for money . . . it's unique in being able to pack so much relevant information into such a small volume, which makes it highly readable

British Medical Association,
on *Fast Facts – Minor Surgery*, 2nd edn,
(First Prize, Primary Health Care, BMA Book Awards 2008)

This short textbook provides a quickstop guide to STIs . . . it's handy for both medical students and allied healthcare professionals

British Medical Association,
on *Fast Facts – Sexually Transmitted Infections*, 2nd edn
(Commended, Public Health Care, BMA Book Awards 2008)

www.fastfacts.com

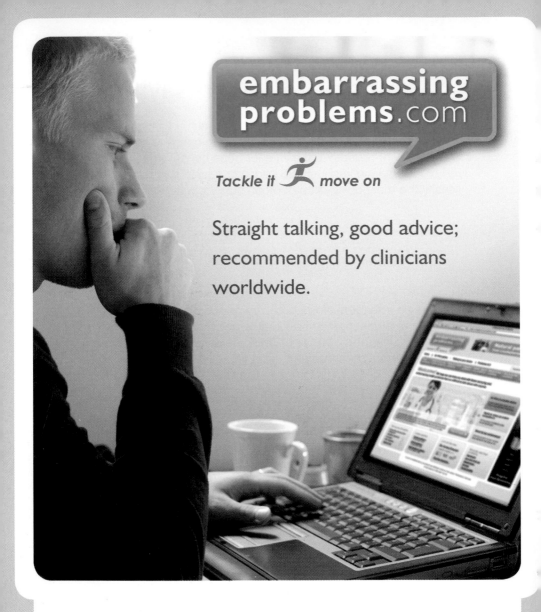